The Metabolism Solution

The NEW way to lose weight

By Lisa Lynn

with Vira Mamchur Schwartz

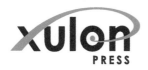

xulon PRESS

Dedicated to all who have struggled with their weight, trying diet after diet, fasting, even starving themselves as well as over-exercising only to gain even more weight. It is my personal mission to help you lose weight and keep it off for life. *The Metabolism Solution* will radically transform your whole life, not just your body. You'll live a happier, healthier, and leaner life—so you can do what God sent you here for.

With Deep Heartfelt Gratitude

It's fitting that this book is called *The Metabolism Solution* because it contains the solution to all your weight loss problems. My intention in writing it is to pass on what I've learned through my own struggles and studies, and to pass on the blessings I've received.

All of the glory goes to God, as He is my strength and inspiration. I want to thank Him for giving me this opportunity to help so many people. As always He guided me through the process.

Thank you also to my editor Vira for displaying dignity and grace under pressure while writing this book, to Frankie, an angel sent from above, for putting it all together, and to my support team/prayer warriors (you know who you are) for sharing my passion and, most of all, for inspiring me to reach further and share more of myself in order to help you succeed. I could not have done it without your support and prayers.

Thank you Mom and Dad for giving me life. Thanks especially to you, Mom, for being my best cheerleader and picking me up every time I fell down.

Thank you Jeff for being such a loving husband even when I didn't deserve it and for loving me no matter what—especially through the darkest hours of my food withdrawal and endless hours of overwork following my life's mission. I couldn't have done it without you.

Thank you Kiana and Kyle. I cherish you; your love and joy and happiness brighten my life and I am grateful for you. You make every day full of life and you always provide me with great food content, not to mention always being good sports about eating your vegetables.

I am extremely grateful and thank God for my best friends, my dogs, who sat with me at my feet every minute of every day writing this book and provided me with unconditional love and constant kisses.

Thank you Grandma and Grandpa for teaching me how to cook delicious tasting food and showing me that yes, food is love.

I'm grateful also to the ministry at Faith Church, particularly Pastor Frank who always knows how to keep my passion in line with God's word and inspires me to keep fighting the good fight. Nothing is greater than our God and any battle we face is no match for God's grace.

Loads of gratitude goes to all of the supporters, all of you who have selflessly shared your stories with me. You inspired me to write this book. Each and every one of you touches me more than you know.

I am grateful to my physical body for carrying me through life and for staying strong and healthy which allowed me to work on my mission every single day and I never take that for granted for one minute.

Finally I'd like to thank my Grandmother Mary Fabrizio, whose courageous battle with pancreatic cancer sparked and fueled my passion and commitment to health and weight loss, and my Grandmother Hannah Smith, who struggled with diabetes and ultimately lost her leg from diabetes complications and never let it slow her down.

Stay Strong, Live Fearlessly, and Be Blessed with Vibrant Health!

Contents

One

HOW I MADE MYSELF FAT AND WHAT I LEARNED

Few struggles frustrate as much as those with weight loss. I know. I'm a recovering compulsive overeater and have struggled with food cravings since childhood. I am the child of two alcoholics, who themselves came from generations of addicts 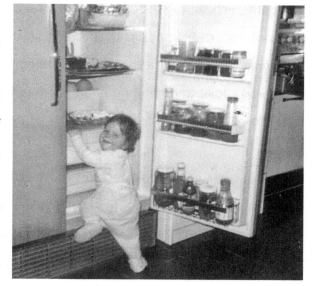 (specifically, but not limited to alcoholism). Looking back at my life now, I feel I was born physically damaged which left me anxious, prone to depression and faulty thinking. Most importantly, spiritually void. When I think of those very early years I remember three things very clearly; the loneliness, feeling unloved, and unsafe. As an adult, I can see that my poor parents struggled so badly with their own addictions, just trying to stay alive, that they had nothing left to give me. Subsequently, as a child, I was left to parent myself. Growing up with an alcoholic father meant I always had to compete with the bottle, leaving me to feel like I wasn't good enough or worthy of his love. To this day I still struggle with not feeling good enough.

It could have been worse however. At least I had a roof over my head and no unexplainable bruises, but it was bad. The emotional lessons I took from my childhood were more devastating than I ever realized at the time. I became the *good* survivor, the "I'll do it myself" girl from an early age. Even when I didn't know how to take care of myself, I managed. I hid the fear and my feelings of unworthiness. I learned how to smile all the time, even when dying on the inside, and kept this up well into adulthood.

It was only thanks to my Mom's decision to get sober (over 40 years ago) following a 12-step program that I had my first inkling of hope. With her new found sobriety she decided to send me to a private Christian school. This was no easy feat as we were just about flat broke. It was there that for the first time I truly felt God's love. I felt safe, fulfilled, and whole.

As a child, food became my reward, my comfort, and my savior. I made the seemingly innocent decision to eat to appease my feelings of anger, frustration, and longing to cover up how uncomfortable physically, emotionally and spiritually I was inside. My childhood quick fix of overeating created a long-term problem where I became overly self-reliant and did not trust God's love and healing. I had food and I had myself. I learned how to feed the hungry heart to numb painful feelings instead of dealing with them head on. Food was my drug of choice.

As an adult, I look back on those painful memories and realize that those childhood experiences, as horrible as they were at the time, shaped me into who I am today. It is only through experiences from which you grow and become the awesome spiritual being God intends you to be. This process, this realization, takes time. With God's help you can overcome anything no matter how big it may seem at the time. Nothing is bigger than our God. God was not the center of my life initially and He certainly wasn't the center of my parents' lives during their alcoholic days. If food, alcohol, exercise – any addiction, becomes the center of your world you are in trouble. In my own spiritual healing I've learned to forgive myself and others, as well as have faith. There is a direct correlation between physical fitness and spiritual fitness.

My father died a horrific death from lung cancer two years ago as an active alcoholic and compulsive smoker. He left behind a legacy of alcoholism and addiction that still affects our family to this day. At the end, he was scared to die. Despite how badly he was suffering he was afraid he wasn't forgiven. How well I remember our last conversation; "Daddy, you don't have to be brave for us and you don't need to suffer anymore. Not only do we love you, but God loves you and your sins have already been forgiven through His son Jesus. You can rest knowing that you are His child and as long as you believe on Him and ask for forgiveness your earthly suffering can transform into a heavenly celebration." The chaplain gave him his last rights and he died the next morning, peacefully.

While tragic and painful, this experience will always be one of my fondest memories with my dad. How joyful to know that I was able to bring him to the Lord in such a peaceful way. And to this day know that even through a lifetime of alcoholism, smoking, and all the ungodliness that follows, God still loved him, just as he does all of us today. He is constantly teaching us that every health and life issue we face; including weight loss, is physically, mentally and spiritually rooted and that we must address all three aspects for true healing to take place. Through that pain, through that blackness, through that tragedy, God loves us.

How can my struggles and mistakes, mentally and spiritually, help you? Well, thanks to my own experiences and struggles with weight, I have learned what the most successful method for fast and guaranteed weight loss is. I have studied and tried just about every weight loss program out there. None of them worked for me. I became vegetarian, meticulously counted calories, religiously kept a food journal, and exercised until I couldn't raise my arm to hold a book—but I only gained weight. If you are one of the lucky ones who have a fast metabolism and never crave the wrong food, stop reading now. If you're like me and struggle with a dead metabolism and have to work at losing weight, then this book will change your life forever.

If you want to lose weight by tomorrow, forget everything you've ever learned and start this plan. What makes *The Metabolism Solution* different? It has a different approach. No guilting, no shaming, no scaring. All food is good food and all exercise is better than none, but there is a method to it, a scientific approach that leaves out "opinions" that trip you up. More of anything isn't better, *better* is better. Why waste your time on dieting and weight loss plans that only tell you what you want to hear? Why waste time on empty promises when you can get results fast?

I have been where you are. Me, a fitness expert. I used to think my clients would not want to hear that. But I was wrong. Not only do I have a slow metabolism due to hyperthyroidism, but I love to eat. My weight struggle was a losing battle until I learned the secret to boosting my metabolism. It is my personal mission to share what I have learned to help you lose the weight you want to feel better and look better. I want to teach you *The Metabolism Solution* so you can keep the weight off for life.

You can do it. When your food is in order, your whole life will be in order. It's worth every ounce of effort you need to put into it. Living *The Metabolism Solution* has not just helped me lose weight; it has changed my body and helped me be happier. Yes, happier. No more do I wake up every day crying and feeling hopeless because I can't control my weight. By letting go of any anxious negative thoughts and surrendering to the process, you too can lose one pound every day until you reach your goal. I guarantee that if you follow *The Metabolism Solution* and stick to it, it works 100 percent of the time.

NOW IS THE TIME TO CHANGE YOUR LIFE FOREVER

Do you want to lose one pound a day? *The Metabolism Solution* is the way to get into the best shape of your life, guaranteed. It's as simple as just making a decision. Making the decision to change. Sounds so easy, doesn't it? When you decide that you're sick and tired of being sick and tired, then and only then, are you ready to make the necessary changes needed to lose weight for life. Deciding - that's the first step.

My story begins with excuses. Sound familiar? I thought that losing weight was for everyone else but not me, the woman who helps thousands of people radically transform their own bodies fast. I thought that because of my hypothyroidism which kept my metabolism at a snail's pace, that I had to starve myself and work out like a crazy woman for hours every day, seven days a week (at the expense of a happier life—ironically, because I was trying to make myself happier by feeling better by losing weight). I tried every diet from the caveman's to South Beach to Atkins to high-carb to low-carb—you name it. I became a vegetarian for a while in a last-ditch attempt to control my growing weight. I would starve myself and

> **THE SCALE IS NOT YOUR GOD.**

then binge on all that I'd been missing. I even joined Overeaters Anonymous. And finally, I told myself that there was nothing more for me to do and I had to learn to accept myself the way I was. I received the same advice from a therapist, "learn to love yourself the way you are." Could I forgive myself for not being a size 6? Possibly. But I just didn't feel good physically. I felt tired all the time and achy, and I was becoming depressed, sad, and desperate. I couldn't even hear God's voice because the self-imposed negative nagging in my head was so loud.

Do you know what I mean? I hated myself. I hated seeing myself in the mirror, and frankly, I was sick and tired of being sick and tired. I fought with food; I struggled to change how I ate and instead became addicted to healthy foods like oatmeal and high-priced whole grains. The more I read, the more I heard about healthy eating for weight loss in the media, the more confused I became. I soon lost all hope. I tried every supplement—even those that made my heart race scarily—I paid any price necessary to see any and all diet gurus about getting my body back on track. People came to *me* for this kind of knowledge and support, yet I couldn't help myself. That's what made it worse. I was a high-level master trainer, a highly regarded sports-nutrition specialist, and I couldn't help myself.

LEARNING FROM THE VERY BEST

Food and I go way back. My mother tells how I couldn't be kept from the chocolate cake in the fridge at the age of 2, as the previous photo proves. And the weight struggle started soon after. Yet somehow I was drawn to a healthy lifestyle. (I thank God for that. What would have happened to me otherwise?) To be brutally honest, I was obsessed with reading and learning everything I could about healthy and fit living because I was so unhappy inside.

Looking back, I truly believed that I was valued only because of the number I reached on the scale and the size I wore. I thought I would just be happier, fit in, and be more successful if I could not pinch that inch on my stomach. It seemed so many of my friends could eat what they wanted and never gain an ounce. They were losing weight. I couldn't stand to look at myself in the mirror. I felt hopeless, convinced that being fit and at a reasonable weight just wasn't for me. The irony is not lost on me that I was just starting out in the fitness business going through my own personal fitness struggle. I studied everything I could get my hands on about losing weight, nutrition, and working out. At my heaviest I topped the scale almost 50 pounds over where I wanted to be. I was helping others, but not myself.

It wasn't until I was asked to work with Dr. Fred Hatfield, an internationally renowned fitness expert, founder of a fitness magazine that is now *Men's Fitness*, and the first person to

> REPLACE FEAR
> WITH **FAITH.**

lift over 1,000 pounds, that I finally had my Aha! Moment. I was obsessively working out for three or more hours when Dr. Hatfield came into the gym in 1991 looking for trainers to work on a study he was running. The test was of the American Heart Association's program and also Cybergenics' (a private company) extreme fat-loss program, which followed the American Heart Association's food pyramid and added 30-minute calisthenics workouts three times a week, against his own ICOPRO (Integrated Conditioning Systems) system, also known as Thermic Force, which was a combination of scientific weight training, other types of training, psychological strategies, nutritional strategies, the targeted use of supplements, and other techniques. At the time I didn't realize that top fitness and nutrition experts as well as elite athletes turned to Dr. Hatfield for help. I had no idea who he was or that my life was about to drastically change.

I readily signed up to work with Dr. Hatfield, but I had my doubts and my fears to cling to. I feared it would work for everyone but me. I thought I knew better, at least for myself. I was so naïve. How could eating more and exercising less (albeit in a more efficient way) cause such drastic changes in my body? No way. If starving myself and spending three hours at the gym wasn't getting me leaner and fitter, how could less exercise possibly work?

Candidates in the study, the men and women, were not just overweight but obese with little to no knowledge about exercise and healthy eating. Watching them finally be able to begin to change their bodies, it became obvious to me that everything I was doing to that point was all wrong. Everything I had learned about weight loss was fear-based. Fear of never being able to eat your favorite food. Fear of being judged. Fear of failure. Dieting and exercising out of fear is no way to succeed.

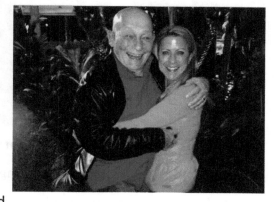

For *The Metabolism Solution* I took everything I learned from Dr. Hatfield and combined it with my own research and experience to finally get myself healthy. I cut my gym time down, focusing on specific, better exercise instead of more reps. I discovered that specific foods could speed my weight loss, boost my metabolism, and that lean protein is necessary. That a simpler plan is the more effective one. And that smart, scientific supplements could truly make a difference without endangering my life. It was hard to make the change, but I am so glad I did.

MIRACLES COME FROM MOTIVATION

I didn't find a miracle in a bottle, but I came close. One of the most frequently asked questions I get every day is about one of my appearances on *The Dr. Oz Show* discussing raspberry ketones. I've gone on Dr. Oz's show repeatedly over the years with fitness tips.

In this particular segment, Dr. Oz used two filled balloons to demonstrate how raspberry ketones, a supplement, can shrink fat cells by affecting our adiponectin (an important protein hormone) levels and tricking our bodies into thinking like a thin person. He

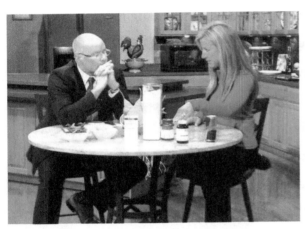

placed the balloons in nitrogen and they shrank to a smaller size. Dr. Oz explained that raspberry ketones can do the same for fat cells and thus make them easier for our bodies to burn. I was there as the expert, to corroborate the segment. Dr. Oz's producers (as well as those of other television shows) call on me when it comes to discussions on fat loss and supplements because they know that I have been studying this topic for 25 years and continue to do so. Through my ongoing studies, I have learned that supplements combined with a thermogenic (fat burning) diet and metabolic-boosting exercises are the only way to get weight off fast. You cannot supplement away a bad diet.

One positive thing I have learned about myself is that I'm coachable. If I'm told to do something, I do it. I don't question or analyze, I just do it. And this brings me to the magnificent Martha Stewart.

One thing people do not know about Martha is that she has incredible "can do" attitude. She never makes excuses. If she doesn't know how to do something, she learns and does it. That remarkable God-given ability got her to where she is today and has taught me

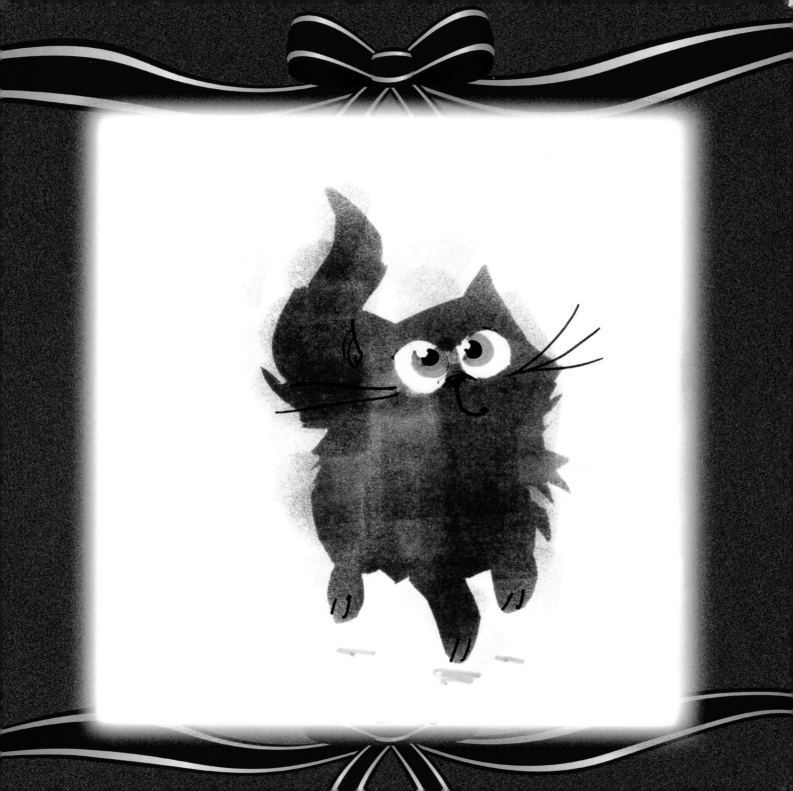

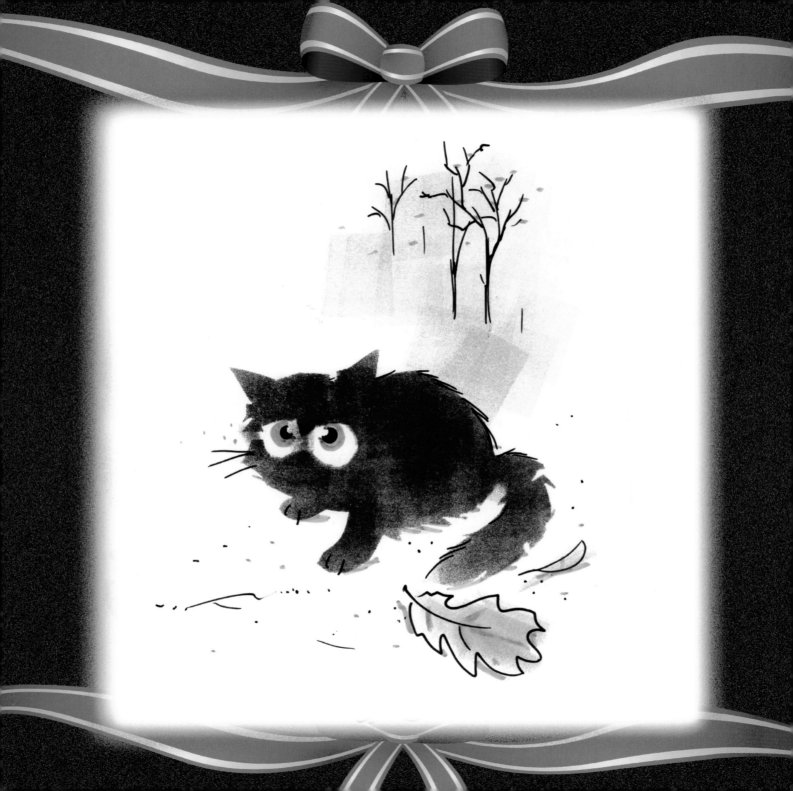

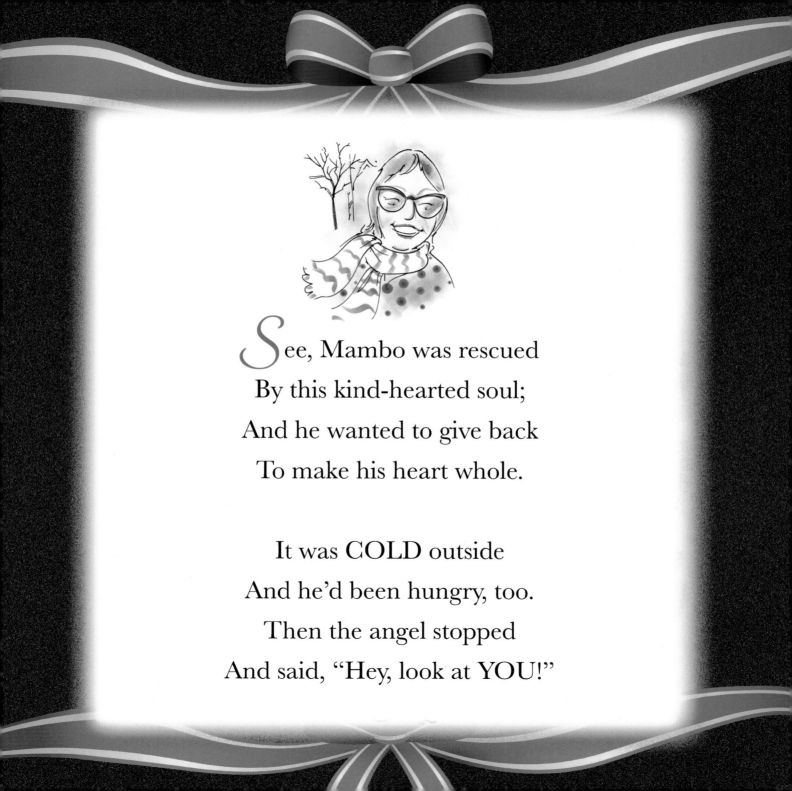

See, Mambo was rescued
By this kind-hearted soul;
And he wanted to give back
To make his heart whole.

It was COLD outside
And he'd been hungry, too.
Then the angel stopped
And said, "Hey, look at YOU!"

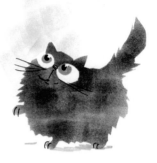

You could use some fresh water,
And how about a hot meal?
Such love and affection,
Could this really be REAL?

He felt so darn happy,
His feet they did prance;
And soon when he walked,
He actually danced!

that anything—and I do mean anything—is possible. Decide to do it and *do* the *do*.

You might think it was at a high-end Pilates studio where I met Martha Stewart. You'd be wrong. I met Martha at a serious body builders' gym at 5:30 in the morning. That's the time when the "I Want-Results" people work out; there's no socializing at that hour. I was working with a client who was a bathing suit model and I would do my metabolic workout

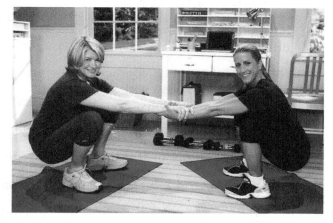

with him at the gym three to four days a week. Martha was there every morning on the treadmill. I was known around the gym as the trainer who got "fast results," and she watched in amazement as I quickly morphed my client's physique into a lean, ready-for-the-beach (and camera) body. One day when he was late for our appointment, Martha asked me for help.

I'll admit, I didn't know who she was. I could tell she was someone special because she had a presence about her. I probably would have been too nervous to speak with her if I had known who she was. Believe it or not, I said I couldn't help her that day because my client was on his way. But Martha didn't give up. The next day she asked me again, and this time I said yes.

I gave Martha the same speech I give all my new clients. Food impacts 80 percent of your results (unless you're over 40 and then it's 90 percent) and exercise is only 20 percent (over 40, 10 percent) of the equation to weight loss. I let Martha in on the weight loss secrets I had learned; to lose weight and fat fast, you need to boost your metabolism so you burn more calories all day long. The key? Drinking a protein shake every day for breakfast (within two hours of waking) to boost your metabolism 25 percent, exercising better (and less), and eating the right kinds of foods.

After working with Martha for a bit, I learned that she had just gone through some difficult emotional times and had recently turned 40 and couldn't lose the weight "no matter what." Martha was frustrated that what she used to do no longer worked, and she was ready for change and results. She admitted that she had never had to watch what she ate; even during her days as a model, she always ate whatever she wanted. But she was learning what every woman learns; when you hit a certain age, what you did in your teens and 20's no longer works. Losing weight is just not that easy the older you get. To be honest, I believe it's harder for people who have never struggled with their weight to lose it later in life—especially around the mid-section—because they don't accept that they have to eat differently and work out differently in order to get their bodies to change.

> **IF MARTHA CAN, SO CAN YOU!**
> - **Have the right tools at your disposal – be it home or away.**
> - **Make fitness your first priority and start every day off with a workout, no matter what.**

Martha had tried several low-calorie diets and still couldn't lose the pounds she wanted to. I explained that a protein shake would be better than starving in the mornings because it would tell her body to *release* fat from storage that could then be burned off as fuel, while just having a coffee for breakfast told her body that food might not be coming so it should hold on to the fat to use for energy later. She was eager to learn all I had to teach and constantly questioned me about everything. I convinced her to switch out the fattening foods and ingredients she ate for simpler ones, and she was stunned when the scale showed the pounds falling away. I explained how to use supplements safely (not my own LynFit brand, but working with Martha was one of the inspirations for starting my own line) to enhance and speed up the fat-burning process, help curb cravings, and block the unwanted carbs from being stored—a trick we all need at times. Lastly, I taught Martha how to work out specifically to boost her sluggish metabolism. I taught Martha everything I teach you in these pages. In return, she called me the "only trainer who got results."

What I admire most about Martha is how incredibly strong, flexible, and unafraid of hard work she is. Her perseverance and determination to do whatever needs to be done is amazing. I have never met a busier person who still manages to get it all done. She prioritizes her fitness because she knows her health and wellness depend on it. It is at the top of her priority list—yes, even above cooking, scrapbooking, and entertaining. Home or away, Martha works out every day.

We used to work out in her kitchen where she originally started her TV show or sometimes in her sun porch where she kept a huge flight cage of singing canaries. Her dogs would gather and watch, and occasionally one would give her a very wet face lick while one of her seven Himalayan cats sat on top her of while she did crunches. Why didn't I mind? The cat added resistance, which helps to strengthen, and it helped guarantee that Martha got her workout in a safe and comfortable environment and in less time. I see it first-hand all the time; those who work out at home get better results in less time because they are much more efficient and consistent since there is no travel to and from the gym. Even when Martha had houseguests she would invite them to join us. She would never miss a workout with me. On Sundays I would meet Martha at her film studio to do cardio, and I would gather as many newspapers as I could, to get her to bike for hours if we weren't able to walk our local beaches (we would always pick up litter as we went).

> I WAS A GUEST on Martha's television show over 50 times. You can find many of these segments on YouTube. Among them I share exercise moves and Martha and I prepare tasty and healthy foods— including the fish recipes in this book (page 209). I'll do whatever it takes to do get people to exercise and that includes cooking for Martha Stewart.

Sometimes I had to bribe Martha with post-workout snacks to get her to finish exercising. I would blend her a protein smoothie, which she drank from a champagne glass naturally, or prepare an egg white breakfast (when a protein shake was on the menu for dinner) so she would finish every single exercise I had planned for the day. I'll do whatever it takes to do get people to exercise and that includes cooking for Martha Stewart. The bottom line: You need a make-it-work attitude and do whatever it takes, as long as it takes.

TURN YOUR I CAN'T INTO I CAN

Let me add one more thing. Martha is not just the person you hear about in the media. She is one of the most honest (brutally honest, to be exact) people you will ever meet. And she is also one of the most considerate. She showed up at my home one Christmas morning with unexpected gifts for my children. I was mortified for Martha to see my messy and very un-Martha like home, but it didn't deter her. She blessed my five-year-old daughter with not one but two Himalayan kittens, saying one would be too lonely. I think it shows how soft and kind she is inside.

Two

THE SUPPLEMENTS THAT BOOST YOUR METABOLISM

I f you remember me from television, it's probably from my appearance on a Dr. Oz episode about the "Miracle in a Bottle." It was a show about the supplement raspberry ketones and how extraordinary it can be in helping weight loss.

The befores and afters shown during the episode that day sparked more public interest in fat-burning supplements than any other episode *ever* according to Dr. Oz staff, and the episode continues to attract more viewers online. The problem is that we only had minutes to discuss raspberry ketones, and we weren't able to say all of the things you need to know before you consider adding the supplement to your weight loss regiment.

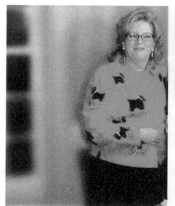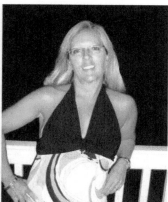

Leslie – Lost a total of 57 pounds!

Real People. Real Results.
While all people are different and individual results will vary, these photos are of LynFit's customers' actual experience.

The show heralded the first time Dr. Oz ever spoke about a "miracle" supplement,

Before taking any supplement, please consult with your doctor, especially if you are taking any other medications. Blood thinners, for instance, are often contraindicated with many supplements. It is important to use supplements responsibly as they may enhance their effects or the effects of your medication when combined. Follow all label directions carefully. Please do not take supplements if you are pregnant or nursing.

raspberry ketones. Raspberries, the fruit, have been around for millennia. They are packed with vitamins and antioxidants and boost the levels of adiponectin, a hormone that helps with fat absorption and regulates metabolism. The higher the levels of adiponectin in the body, the less the fat. Unfortunately, to boost adiponectin levels you would have to eat more raspberries than humanly possible in a day, but modern supplements put all you need in one capsule.

This is where you need to be particularly careful. It's a jungle out there when it comes to purchasing supplements. You need to know your facts before you put down your dollars.

> PROPERLY COMBINED AND IN THE RIGHT AMOUNTS, SUPPLEMENTS RAMP UP A METABOLISM.

And beware of segments on television touting the effectiveness of a particular brand; they are almost always a *paid* commercial and you just don't know it. Buy from a reputable source, and when in doubt, don't!

YOU CANNOT SUPPLEMENT AWAY A BAD DIET

First and foremost, taking a pill will not magically drop you a dress size. You cannot supplement away a bad diet. Nevertheless, weight loss supplements can be very helpful, downright miraculous, when combined with a thermogenic diet and metabolic exercise.

> **THE TOP THREE REASONS DIETS FAIL**
> 1) Hunger/Cravings
> 2) Lack of energy/Not feeling good
> 3) Sluggish metabolisms

Our bodies are designed for a steady supply of varied nutrients and photochemicals. We *need* them in our diets and by following *The Metabolism Solution* you will get an awesomely abundant healthy supply of what your body needs. Losing body fat, however, is a metabolic issue and stubborn body fat likes to decide its own destiny. (See Thermogenic Eating for Radical Weight Loss on page 85 to boost your metabolism). Fat can actually burn itself—if you provide it with specific nutrients. And this is where supplements help—by burning fat and calories *faster*.

My specialty is revving the metabolism, known as metabolic hyping in the fitness world. Metabolic hyping creates an optimal environment for fat loss by helping to lower blood sugar levels and enhancing metabolism—this is the secret to melting fat faster. Metabolic hyping multiplies calorie burn so you burn more calories and fat all day long—exactly what you want if your metabolism is stuck, if you are over 40, or if you are plagued with a sluggish metabolism. No one eats perfectly, and you cannot spend every waking hour at the gym. It's next to impossible to lower blood sugar when you are inundated

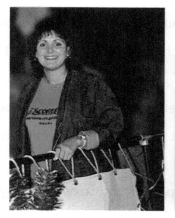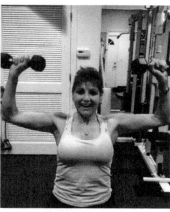

Lynn – Lost 20 Pounds Right Away!

Real People. Real Results.
While all people are different and individual results will vary, these photos are of LynFit's customers' actual experience.

with constant cravings and hunger. Food is in our faces 24 hours a day, seven days a week.

Recent discoveries in the field of weight management and obesity suggest that dieting and restricting calories (depriving the body of nutrients) decreases a body's ability to burn fat. Your body thinks it needs to hold on to fat for future use when it is deprived. Yet we all know that reducing calories is the only proven way to lose weight. So how do you do it? Supplements. When combined with a thermogenic diet (see Thermogenic Eating for Radical Weight Loss on page 85 for more), supplements can optimize

SMART SUPPLEMENTS CAN HELP BREAK THROUGH PLATEAUS.

the metabolism, shifting it into high gear—which is where fat begins to be burned and melt off your body.

But here's the catch (and there always seems to be one); supplements work better when combined. This is what makes my brand of LynFit supplements different from every other

supplement out there. I've combined a matrix of tested ingredients as opposed to a single-ingredient formula. Your body never adapts or gets immune to what you are taking and keeps your metabolism guessing, which causes it to accelerate. I took the guesswork out of supplementing and combined the most effective, research-based, time-tested ingredients in exactly the amounts your body needs. Why settle for one ingredient when you get the most comprehensive supplements system in three LynFit formulas?

Most overweight people (those who struggle to lose weight) suffer with genuine hunger—real gnawing hunger—which is often caused by nutrient deficiencies brought on by aging, stress, and lack of a nutritious diet as well as the body's inability to absorb certain nutrients. Thus, you lose weight at a slower rate, struggle with severe cravings and abnormal hunger, and have an overall lack of energy which keeps you from following a fitness plan. Scientific studies show that using supplements at specific times in specified amounts, known as smart supplementing or nutrient partitioning, is the solution. Supplements can help solve the issues that derail our diets. They can instantly help eliminate emotional urges to eat and stress-eating binges, control your appetite, decrease after-meal sugar levels, and block fat and carbs from being absorbed so they can't be stored as fat. Supplements should always be safe and, not only should they help you achieve your weight loss goals, they should also be *functional*. Supplements "solve" a problem by providing your body with the needed nutrients and assist your body in the process; they don't do it for you.

THE STANDARD FOR SAFE AND SUCCESSFUL SUPPLEMENTING

With supplement sales reaching over $30 billion in the United States alone, it is a big business. Almost half of all Americans take or have taken at one time some kind of supplement. Technically not considered a "drug," dietary supplements go through different testing than your standard medications. The Food and Drug Administration oversees all supplements under the Federal Drug, Food and Cosmetic Act as amended by the Dietary Supplement Health and Education Act of 1994 (DSHEA).

The Natural Products Association, a nonprofit founded in 1936 dedicated to the natural products industry, was a key player in DSHEA's passage. The organization set up a GMP (Good Manufacturing Practices) seal program and since 2010 all manufacturers fall under GMP regulations, as established by the FDA. To earn a GMP seal, products go through a third-party GMP-certification program, which includes third-party inspections of the factories as well as specific documentation. A GMP seal means the product has been made using the industry's best practices and met a high level of control. These include identifying all ingredients (only those federally sanctioned can be used), their strength, testing for contaminants, and additional testing for final products.

The Office of Dietary Supplements was established and authorized with the passage of DSHEA. Its role is to promote research of supplements, aggregate the research and studies, and serve in an advisory capacity to the directors of the National Institute of Health as well as the FDA commissioner regarding supplements.

The FDA is supposed to ensure that supplement labels are not misleading, that no medical claims are made (hence the wording; "This statement has not been evaluated by the U.S. Food and Drug Administration (FDA). This product is not intended to diagnose, treat, cure, or prevent any disease."), and that GMP standards are met. Once on the market, the FDA tracks a product by research and following consumer complaints of side effects to deduce if a product should be removed due to safety concerns. Supplement manufacturers are responsible for making sure that their products are safe.

The U.S. Pharmacopeial Convention (USP) is another organization that has developed international standards that include supplement identity, strength, quality, and purity. Medicines and food ingredients also must meet these standards. The USP has been setting standards for vitamins and minerals since its inception in 1820. Only products meeting the organizations most stringent criteria receive the USP label.

But who decides how much, say, vitamin B you need a day? That would be the Food and Nutrition Board (FNB), which is part of the National Academy of Sciences. Part of the Institute of Medicine, the FNB began in 1940 and set the first nutritional standards in 1941. These standards were originally known as the Recommended Daily Allowance (RDA) and

IF YOUR GOAL IS WEIGHT LOSS, YOU NEED THESE SUPERSTAR INGREDIENTS IN YOUR SUPPLEMENTS.

currently go by the Dietary Reference Intake (DRI). These determine the amount of nutrients needed daily to meet the dietary needs of 97.5 percent of all healthy people. New DRIs are currently being reviewed by several panels of independent experts; the process is expected to take at least 5 years. How do you decide what to take? Follow an expert's advice and base it on your needs. Here are my superstars.

SUPERCHARGE YOUR METABOLISM WITH SUPERSTAR INGREDIENTS

From the millions of supplements out there, there is a group of ingredients that any reputable supplement claiming to help in weight loss must include. I call these the superstar ingredients. Toxicity of these nutrients is extremely rare in healthy adults, but it doesn't hurt to be cautious. Never exceed suggested dosages, take a day off every two weeks—but not on a cheat day, as that's where you need it most.

B Vitamins

The B vitamin family is always important when it comes to taking supplements because of their ability to help metabolize (breakdown food to convert it to energy); they are crucial for any weight loss program. Emotional, mental, and physical stress demand more B's. Without enough B's, you'll feel tired, stressed, and irritable—the exact things you don't want when you're trying to lose weight. That's why it's best to combine the B vitamins in a weight loss formula the way LynFit does.

B1 (Thiamine), B2 (Riboflavin), B3 (Niacin), B5 (Pantothenic Acid), B6 (Pyridoxine), and B12 (Cobalamin) are water-soluble vitamins (excess amounts pass easily in urine) found in the following foods—but not limited to—unprocessed foods (processed foods deplete our bodies), whole grains, potatoes, bananas, chili peppers, and beans. The best source for B12 is animal protein. I'm not suggesting you eat all these foods, by the way; they're just a good natural source and unfortunately B vitamins come from all of the foods you need to limit when trying to lose weight and force your body to burn fat.

> MORE ISN'T BETTER, BETTER IS BETTER.

Workouts and stress deplete B vitamins big time. And who isn't stressed these days? If you live with anxiety, you need B vitamins more than ever. When you nourish your body with what it needs, cravings begin to diminish. B vitamins aren't just good for your metabolism they are also good for heart health. B's make red blood cells which are responsible for carrying oxygen into your body's tissues, making these vitamins essential for a stress-free body that's tightly toned and cellulite-free.

L-Carnitine

L-Carnitine is an essential amino acid that has been studied since 1937. It is naturally produced in the body, found in red meat, and best known for its ability to transport fat into

> SUPPLEMENTING IS A BETTER WAY TO GET NUTRIENTS BECAUSE THEY ARE BETTER ABSORBED AND WITHOUT ADDED CALORIES, SUGAR, OR FAT.

cells so that fat can be burned easier for energy, a process known as fatty oxidation. If you lack natural L-Carnitine, you have a hard time turning fat into fuel and can suffer from muscle weakness, soreness, and other serious conditions. Supplementing with L-Carnitine can help burn fat and give more energy during a workout while helping to prevent muscle soreness.

A study published in *Food and Chemical Toxicology* (September 2011) included two groups of mice on a high-fat, weight-gaining diet. One of the groups was supplemented with L-Carnitine, the other a placebo. When compared, the L-Carnitine group gained considerably *less* weight. There was some concern that taking L-Carnitine could lead to heart problems in humans however. A meta-analysis study published in Mayo Clinic Proceedings in 2013, looked at *13 different studies* on L-Carntine's effects and concluded that it is, in fact, helpful against heart disease.

Choline

> TAKING SUPPLEMENTS DAILY CAN HELP YOU LOSE WEIGHT WITHOUT STARVING. AND THEY CAN PROVIDE THE ADDED BENEFIT OF BOOSTING YOUR METABOLISM SO YOU BURN MORE FAT FASTER.

Only recently classified as a vitamin, choline is part of the B-complex vitamin family. It is found in eggs, seafood, wheat, and peanuts. It too, is made by our bodies, but to increase its benefits you would have to eat too many fatty foods, so nutrient supplementation is the preferred way so that you eat less fat in order to burn fat. Taking choline as a supplement also allows for higher accuracy in correct dosage. When you are short on choline, you may feel week, lack mental clarity, and feel in a depressed mood. It's best known for balancing out blood fat levels, especially cholesterol—but it doesn't discriminate—and increases the rate of fat burning.

Inositol

This vitamin, also known as B8, is another member of the B-complex family and can be found in nuts, beans, wheat, cantaloupe, and oranges. It's best known for boosting metabolic processes, such as breaking down fats so they are burned as fuel and not stored, as well as for controlling estrogen, a hormone critical for fat loss and general health. Inositol is needed for proper heart and brain functioning and helps cells damaged by disease or overuse of antibiotics, and is also used for depression, recovering addicts, anxiety, and stress. (*Note: Many who struggle with weight loss are anxious and/or depressed, which causes overeating and thereby deficiencies in these nutrients. This can create a vicious cycle of overeating which makes it near impossible to lose weight.*) The University of Pittsburgh Medical Center found inositol a generally safe supplement based on a study in March 2009. Choline and inositol combined are the super team; together they produce lecithin, an essential fatty acid that plays a key role in transporting nutrients into cells. Lecithin makes fat loss easier by increasing your fat-burning metabolism.

Choline and Inositol combined are the super team; together they produce lecithin, an essential fatty acid that plays a key role in transporting nutrients into cells. Lecithin makes fat loss easier by increasing your fat-burning metabolism.

L-Methionine

This is an essential amino acid we need to consume from proteins like eggs, fish, Brazil nuts, and cereal grains because our bodies do not produce it. L-methionine is needed to create creatinine, which give muscles energy for movement. When it comes to meeting your body's metabolic requirements, supplementing is the preferred method as eating these foods would yield ultra-high-calorie amounts stopping weight loss. With a supplement, your body absorbs the exact amount needed to fuel your metabolism.

L-methionine is known for its ability to break down fats and remove heavy metals from the body, which aside from slowing down your metabolism can also cause all kinds of diseases. It is especially helpful in helping your body detox from overuse of acetaminophen.

Linoleic Acid

Part of the Omega-6 family of fats that is needed for optimal functioning of the body—specifically with regards to weight loss and metabolism—Linoleic Acid is an essential polyunsaturated fatty acid. Not made by the body, it can be found in safflower oil, sunflower oil, pine nuts, corn oil, soy beans, pecans, Brazil nuts, cottonseed, sesame oil, flax seed, walnuts, and canola oil. It's used in supplements to reduce fat and to prevent fat from returning. A study published in the *Journal of Physiology and Biochemistry* in 2005 found that healthy adults who took the supplement for two years lost weight and reduced body fat mass regardless of diet.

Raspberry Ketones

Raspberry ketones have been used safely for centuries to help alleviate gastrointestinal disorders, respiratory disorders, diabetes, and general purification of the blood, general discomfort from

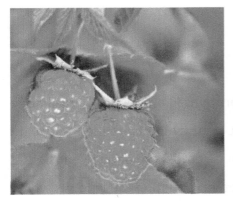

heavy periods, motion sickness, sore throat, skin rashes, and fluid retention—to name just a few. It wasn't until Dr. Oz and I discussed ketones and how they "trick your body into acting like a thin person" on his talk show that raspberry ketones became a household name. Raspberry ketones is the most-searched topic on the Dr. Oz website and the most searched supplement on the internet. News outlets reported how after the Dr. Oz segment, stores couldn't keep enough raspberry ketones on the shelves.

While I could only touch upon the benefits of Raspberry Ketones during my three-minute segment with Dr. Oz, I want to give you the whole story. Here's the skinny (pun intended) on all you need to know.

During my television appearance, Dr. Oz mentioned that he found raspberry ketones appealing because they are natural and "smell nice." Raspberries look fresh and wholesome and their scent is used in lotions, perfumes, candles, and as a flavoring in all kinds of products. The term "ketone" has powerful associations with popular low-carb regimens like the Atkins Diet, which forces your body to burn its own fat for fuel and, thus, produces ketones. Those ketones are not the same as raspberry ketones. What's the difference? Raspberry ketones are compounds that give raspberries their distinct aroma and unique flavor. Even though raspberry ketones have become known as "the miracle in a bottle," there is no magic bullet for weight loss. No pill on its own will make you lose weight in a healthy fashion. But combined with the right regiment, raspberry ketones are perhaps as close as we currently come to being that very miracle in a bottle.

> **STOP** TAKING IT IF YOU DON'T SEE RESULTS IN **2** WEEKS.

I have used raspberry ketones throughout my whole career to help people lose weight fast; to jump start a stalled diet, to lose that last 5 to 10 pounds, and to break through a plateau. Raspberry ketones are one of the main reasons I decided to write this book. The supplement continues to get much attention on television talk shows and I still receive thousands of emails asking me about them. I began using raspberry ketones decades ago when I hit my own weight plateau. The supplement has been approved by the FDA as "generally safe" since 1965. Those last 5 to 10 pounds are the hardest to lose and I needed and wanted a catalyst, an accelerator, to get those results faster and break through the barriers and melt the fat that didn't want to budge. Reaching that plateau after losing and losing and suddenly getting stuck is disheartening. It's easy to get anxious and fall back into old habits. If you have struggled with weight loss (and especially if you're over 30), you know exactly what I am talking about. And this is the moment where the big guns are needed.

There are far too many scams out there to get you to buy the miracle in a bottle. Before you make a purchase, remember:

1) Buy quality—you'll need less.
2) Buy natural, pure product from a *reputable source*, preferably one you know.
3) Quality counts or you won't see results.
4) Make sure you know how much to take and when (and why) before you make that purchase.
5) If you don't see results in two weeks, stop. You probably won't receive any benefit. High-quality works fast.

THE 10 THINGS TO KNOW ABOUT RASPBERRY KETONES

1) Raspberry ketones will help you lose fat when combined with a clean diet and exercise
2) Raspberry Ketones will help you burn fat more effectively, especially if you are not overloading your body with fat.
3) Raspberry Ketones will make you feel full so you'll eat less—but you still need to eat less.
4) Raspberry Ketones need to be combined with a spark of caffeine to help jumpstart the fat loss process.
5) Raspberry Ketones must be combined with other fat-burning agents for best results.
6) Raspberry Ketones are not more effective in higher doses. In fact, you forfeit the fat-burning response if you take too much. Stick with the 100 mg of a high-quality Raspberry Ketones supplement for best results and to break through plateaus.
7) Raspberry Ketones will make you feel better, and when you feel better you move more and eat less.
8) Raspberry Ketones will not work if they are not high-quality.
9) Raspberry Ketones are an awesome way to help you lose that last 5 to 10 pounds in fat.
10) Raspberry Ketones are a great addition to a complete fat-burning supplement program as a last step, not the first step.

Raspberry ketones have shown great promise in two studies. One in 2005 published in *Life Sciences*, showed that raspberry ketones helped mice on a high-fat diet lose weight and protected their livers against fatty buildup. A second study in *Planta Medica* in 2010 ascertained that raspberry ketones help activate adiponectin, a hormone regulating fat breakdown.

Forskolin

You may have heard me on *Dr. Oz* talking about this superstar. Forskolin is one of the best kept secrets when it comes to igniting your metabolism. It has two nicknames worth noting; "lightening in a bottle" because it can double your weight loss and the "Flat Belly Flower" because it excels at breaking up stubborn belly fat. Forskolin is a member of the mint and lavender family and is more commonly known as Coleus Forskohli. Scientists are just now confirming its benefits for weight loss, but it has been used by Ayurvedic doctors for thousands of years to treat all kinds of ailments from allergies to asthma to psoriasis to glaucoma to cancer and depression. I love it because of what it does for weight 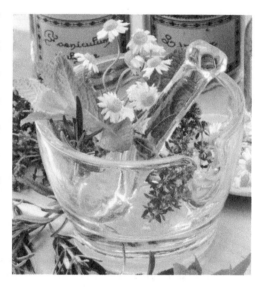 loss. Dr. Oz raved about it; "It really does ignite your metabolism so you lose weight and feel results right away." A 2005 study published in *Obesity Research* found that taking forskolin decreased body fat percentage and fat mass. It works by increasing cAMP, an enzyme that helps with fat breakdown in the body—thermogensis.

While daily calorie reduction is the only proven method to lose weight, it can prove to be a catastrophe for an already sluggish metabolism, which slows down even more. Why? Because your body fears its food (and hence energy) supply is drying up so you immediately begin to lose lean muscle tissue (unless you follow *The Metabolism Solution* thermogenic eating plan detailed in Chapter 4 which starts on page 85) and store fat. Forskolin combined with its fellow superstar ingredients forestalls this metabolic disaster by ensuring that you have as many thermogenic—metabolic boosting—engines going as you possibly can. Why take a chance and risk not losing weight when you're working so hard?

Forskolin is best at protecting this hard-earned lean muscle tissue while you are restricting calories to lose weight, and it also aids in the production of thyroid hormones, helping to keep your thyroid regulated while you lose weight. Preserving lean muscle tissue and keeping your thyroid revved is critical for lasting weight loss, especially if you already have a sluggish thyroid.

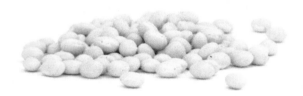

White Kidney Bean Extract

We have become a society with a carb-heavy diet. You do need to watch those breads, pastas, and other starches. But wouldn't it be great if you could take something that would stop those carbs—when you do indulge—from turning straight into sugar and then fat? White Kidney Bean (also known as cannellini beans) Extract, Phaseolus Vulgaris—from the common bean plant—may be the answer.

Taken before a meal, White Kidney Bean Extract works by blocking the digestion of complex carbohydrates; instead of breaking them down, complex carbs pass through the body or are used by the colon as food for healthy bacteria. It is known specifically as

PHASE 2 WHITE KIDNEY BEAN EXTRACT

DEVELOPED BY **New Jersey-based Pharmachem Laboratories Inc., Phase 2 is a specific brand used in many supplements, including those by LynFit. It is a highly concentrated extract made from a portion of the white kidney bean using a proprietary process that assures its potency and purity. Only non-genetically modified beans are used and virtually all impurities are removed. Note that scientific studies regarding white kidney bean extract have only been done using Phase 2, not generic beans.**

alpha-amylase inhibitor isoform 1, a starch inhibitor, and can be found in any bean, but white kidney beans contain the most of this chemical and have become

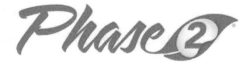

synonymous with the supplement name. It is thought to help against colon cancer as well.

White Kidney Bean Extract taken in conjunction with a reduced calorie diet may help in weight loss. Thirteen different clinical studies show its potential effectiveness in blocking starch absorption. A 2007 study published in the *International Journal of Medical Sciences* used a double-blind, placebo-controlled group and found that those taking white kidney bean extract lost more weight than those who were on the placebo.

On its own, white kidney bean extract is *not* a magic pill, but combined with a reduced calorie-diet it can make a difference. You can find the same benefit in eating beans which are rich in antioxidants and full of fiber. However, be ready to eat for a while. You'd have to eat so much of the beans to get the benefit found in one supplement that it

> **THE EXACT EXTRACT**
>
> DRIED HERBS crushed into powder can vary from harvest to harvest. Not so an extract. An extract is when an herb is soaked in a liquid to take out certain components; one or more of its components is always in a standardized, guaranteed amount. The liquid can be evaporated to create a powder that can then be used in capsules or tablets. Extracts are far more potent and stay fresh longer than drops or other forms of ingredients. I prefer extracts because you get a more nutrient-consistent dose.

would defeat the purpose of helping you lose weight. As with all supplements, but especially here, quality matters. You want the highest quality of white kidney bean extract you can afford. The higher the quality may also offset potential unpleasant side effects of flatulence and diarrhea.

Guggulsterone

This plant steroid is found in the guggul plant, a flowering plant that grows from Northern

Africa to Central Asia and has long been used in Indian Aryuvedic medicine. The gum resin from the plant is used to treat arthritis, atherosclerosis, and other skin diseases as well as high cholesterol. Guggolsterone is thought to be an anti-inflammatory and believed to have an antibacterial property that helps with acne.

Guggul works for weight loss by affecting the thyroid. The thyroid is critical to weight loss. The thyroid's hormones control metabolism and affect thermogenesis. Thyroid hormones can actually stimulate protein synthesis, which is a big plus for bodybuilders and other athletes.

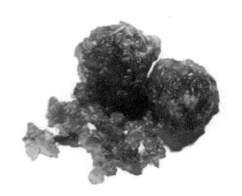

Neither an appetite suppressant nor a stimulant, guggul increases thyroid hormone levels and speeds up metabolism. On a diet, T3 (thyroid hormone) levels decrease slowing down your metabolism as your body receives the signal that it is not getting enough food. When you *increase* your T3 levels, you get better fat loss. A study in 1999 in the April issue of *Current Therapeutic Research* showed guggul's promise for weight loss, helping obese individuals lose significant body fat.

To be effective for weight loss, guggulsterone is best in extract form, not powder form. The brown guggul is far more effective than the yellow. It is also more effective when mixed with other nutrients such as forskolin. It is not to be taken long-term, as guggulsterones can, theoretically, increase your metabolism to such a rate that it is burning up muscles as well as fat. It is important to increase your protein when taking it.

Banaba Leaf

Banaba is a type of crepe myrtle tree with distinct purple flowers that grows in the Philippines and Southeast Asia. It has been used in traditional medicines for centuries, brewed as a tea and used to treat for blood sugar as well as liver and kidney ailments.

If you think of your body as a car, glucose (blood sugar) is the gas. Not enough glucose, you're hungry; full tank—you're ready to go. How much glucose you have in your body is the deciding factor on whether to burn or store fat. The hormone insulin, created in your pancreas, moves the glucose to your body's cell to be used for energy. If you are eating too many carbs, your pancreas goes overboard producing insulin, which tells your body you need energy and therefore stores the glucose as fat. This can easily turn into a vicious cycle.

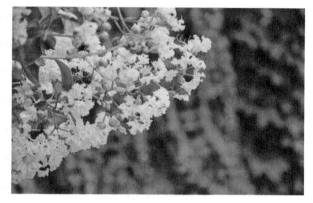

Various clinical studies have shown banaba leaf to be useful in lowering blood sugar levels in those with typically high levels and to be useful in weight loss where high blood sugar has caused obesity. Banaba works because it contains corsolic acid, which works like insulin in the body to lower glucose levels. A 1999 Japanese study published in the *Journal of Nutritional Science and Vitaminology* found mice given banaba leaf lowered their weight and body fat. Another study in a 2003 issue of *the Journal of Ethnopharmacology* found that banaba lowered glucose levels by 30 percent for human test subjects with Type II diabetes.

Chocolate Bean Powder

I just love the name. Anything chocolate works for me. Chocolate Bean Powder is an amazing ingredient that makes us feel good. Go ahead and google it. All are in agreement that it is a superfood. When we feel good, we eat better and crave less, saving lots of calories and hours in the gym. Chocolate bean powder, *Theobroma cacoa*, which translates to "cacoa, food of the gods," is the main ingredient in everyday chocolate. The reason we initially crave chocolate isn't because of the sugar (although that follows later), but because it raises the level of serotonin, the feel-good hormone in our brains. And serotonin, aside from improving mood, helps with sleep and appetite suppression.

Chocolate Bean Powder has been used to treat high blood pressure, cancer, and other

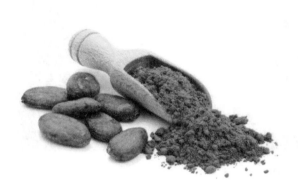

degenerative diseases. You'll find more antioxidant flavinoids in chocolate bean powder than in just about any other natural food. And cacao provides more magnesium than any other food source. The raw cacao bean, from which the powder is made, is estimated to include 30 phytochemicals aside from magnesium. These include calcium, potassium, sodium, sulfur, zinc, and copper. These beans have been revered enough to be used as currency by ancient societies.

Of special note: You'll find caffeine and theobromine in chocolate bean powder. These thermogenic compounds are fat burners. A study in 2005 published in *Nutrition* concluded that taking cocoa can help with weight loss (decreasing fat) by reducing fat production and increasing fat burning, thermogenesis, in white adipose tissue. (Thermogenesis occurs when you use more calories to digest a food than found in the food itself.)

Remember: This is not your standard chocolate. Chocolate, milk chocolate and others

GOD
MADE CHOCOLATE

used in candy, includes cocoa butter, sweeteners and many other additives and is so highly processed that most of the benefits are removed. This is another expensive but highly effective ingredient that needs to be of the utmost highest quality in order to be good for you and help you lose fat. Cocoa needs to be de-fatted and purified (to remove any lead or heavy metals that may be present) in an expensive process to help with fat loss. You cannot eat high-grade chocolate and get these benefits. You'd be adding to much fat when trying to burn fat. It is not the same. Sorry, eating a chocolate bar a day will not help you lose weight.

Omega-3 Fatty Acids

My specialty is metabolic resistance, which means I specialize in getting the most sluggish metabolisms to move faster so more calories are burned and more excess fat is shed. The way Omega-3's can burn belly fat amazes me. Dr. Barry Sears, father of the Zone Diet, once said about Omega-3's; "It's as close to a miracle drug as I'll ever see in my lifetime." I totally agree. Fish oil, which includes cod liver oil, is a

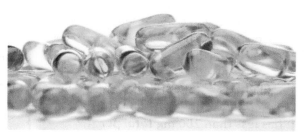

significant source of the Omega-3 fatty acids EPA (Eicosapentaeonic Acid) and DHA (Docosahexaenoic Acid). These fatty acids have more documented health benefits than I could possibly list. They include: weight loss; blood sugar balance; improved cholesterol balance; reduced inflammation; increased blood flow; reduced blood pressure; lower blood fats like triglycerides; reduced rates of heart disease and arteriosclerosis; improved immunity; improved brain function including memory; improved sleep, vision, and nerve health; improvement in psychiatric disorders; and prevention of cancers—particularly breast, colon, and prostate. Improved blood flow and reduced inflammation are of particular interest to anyone who plays sports and works out. Taking Omega-3 allows for

EVERY PERSON AND ANIMAL SHOULD SUPPLEMENT WITH OMEGA-3

faster recovery so you can train more frequently. And while it is naturally abundant in fish, we, especially in the United State, do not eat enough seafood. Fish three to four times a week is great, but it would not even deliver the amount of omega-3 we need.

What fascinates me the most is how Omega-3 can help burn belly fat—but only if you are taking a high-quality Omega-3 with the right ratio of EPA and DHA. This ratio of EPA and DHA is important not only for vanity reasons (shrinking the "spare tire") but because belly fat has a life of its own. What makes belly fat different is that it secretes hormones that are dangerous to our whole health—not just our waistlines.

Omega-3's, and the best come from fish oil (yet they should not have any fishy taste or smell), are necessary to just about all bodily functions. Omega-3's are the ultimate anti-inflammatory, and inflammation is often what leads to disease. Fish oil has been shown to improve Alzheimer's patients' speech, help with joint pain for those suffering from arthritis, and decrease the effects of asthma. Not all Omega-3s are created equal, however. Did you know that most store-bought Omega-3 supplements have saturated fats and toxins in them? Studies have shown that supplementing with high-quality Omega-3 fish oil (Fish, not from a plant; plant sources just don't measure up) can cause weight loss because it

> ### THE IMPORTANT DHA-TO-EPA RATIO
>
> The amount of fish oil you take isn't nearly as important as the ratio of DHA to EPA *in* that fish oil. This ratio varies wildly by brand and quality. When looking at the DHA and EPA content of the fish oil, you want at least 500 mg of each. This is usually listed on the back label.
>
> To make things simple, the total milligrams of EPA and DHA should be 1,000. I've found fish oil in stores that has less than 200 mg *total* per capsule—that's nowhere near enough to make a difference and it's usually from a poor-quality source. On the other hand, anything over 600 mg each DHA and EPA per capsule is pretty potent stuff, it's sometimes called "pharmaceutical grade."
>
> If your brand doesn't list the EPA and DHA content at all (it's not required by law), then walk away and do not buy it. If it's not listed I'm led to believe that the product is of such poor quality that they're ashamed to.

helps lower your insulin levels making it easier for your body to shed excess (or forces your body to release stored fat) fat specifically from the stomach, hips, and thighs. It also improves body composition even when you have a very poor diet.

Of course I suggest that everyone eat a diet rich in fish, lean meat, vegetables, and fruits along with *small* amounts of nuts and seeds, with as little starch and refined sugar as possible. However, if you simply refuse to change your diet, then I highly recommend you take fish oil. In fact, it's even more important for you as you need to offset the effects of a poor diet. It's the least expensive thing you can do to improve your health besides working out. It's also inexpensive compared to the high cost of junk food and the toll it takes on your body, and it's super easy and will go a long way towards counteracting the not-so-good choices we all make.

In 2009, *Obesity Reviews* published a study showing that obese test animals given Omega-3's reduced their body fat. Another study published in the journal *Appetite* (November 2008) ascertained that Omega-3's helped their human volunteers feel more satiated after eating and therefore they were able to lose more weight. The study's authors concluded the participants felt less hunger and felt fuller. A similar study of young adults published in the *International Journal of Obesity* in 2007 found that by including lean or fatty fish or fish oil, participants lost *more* weight—boosted their weight loss—than those who did not include the seafood or fish oil supplement. Also worth noting: A Harvard study in the *Journal of Clinical Endocrinology & Metabolism* from 2013 found that fish oil supplements may help prevent Type 2 Diabetes.

The only significant negative effect of fish oil is that when taken in large doses and combined with drugs like aspirin, it can cause increased bleeding. This doesn't mean you will bleed out from a paper cut, but it could be significant if you incurred a life-threatening injury. This would probably only happen in rare circumstances where you take an extremely large dose *and* combine that with an anti-coagulant like aspirin *and* suffer life-threatening bleeding. If you are having a scheduled surgery, most doctors ask you to stop taking fish oil several days (if not up to two weeks) before any procedure. I think the benefits far outweigh the risks, but that's a decision you must make for yourself. Talk to your doctor.

THE POWER OF PROTEIN: THE ONE THING YOU CAN DO EVERY DAY TO SPEED WEIGHT LOSS

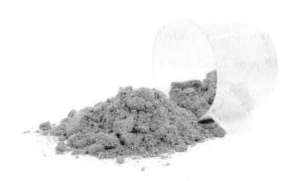

Amino acids. I could write a book on this subject alone. Amino acids as found in protein are the number 1 nutrient we lack—especially women. You would think that with a society that eats so much meat (a key source) this couldn't happen, but there are a lot of variables to consider. For instance, much of our meat is so processed that its nutritional value is undercut if not destroyed. Our bodies cannot digest and utilize the nutrients so we never get the benefits.

The easiest way to gain the protein we so need is via a high-grade whey protein shake. These are microfiltered and already broken down for you so the minute you drink it, all nutrients can be shuttled immediately into your body and used for building lean muscle tissue as well as supporting hair, skin, nails, and hormone regulation. Everyone benefits from the nutrients found in protein whey shakes.

> **STAY AWAY FROM PREMADE/PREPACKAGED SHAKES**
> **THE SECOND they are placed into the containers that sit on store shelves, the shakes begin losing their effectiveness. And lower-quality whey never had any to begin with. Many include far too much sugar. You need high-grade-whet. Follow Martha Stewart's advice: If you cannot buy the quality necessary, save up until you can.**

Protein helps our bodies make tissue and control metabolic, enzymatic, and cellular functions. Amino acids are protein's building blocks and they also are essential to your nervous system, where they help your brain send and receive messages and can be useful against depression and anxiety.

Amino acids are crucial to your body. There are 20 most common types, 10 of these amino acids your body can produce, the remaining 10 need to be ingested either via diet or supplementation daily because they cannot be stored. A protein shake is the easiest way to meet your body's requirements. If your body does not get enough amino acids, it will breakdown living tissue—including organs and muscle—to do so. As you get older, your body's metabolism becomes less efficient—slowing down—and an increase in amino acids can easily help bring you back up to speed.

Many conditions deplete amino acids from the body causing metabolic functions to slow down. Among these: anxiety, depression, aging, and drugs. For instance, many researchers believe that an imbalance in serotonin (a hormone that helps relay messages from one part of the brain to another) is a factor in depression. Our bodies need the essential amino acid L-tryptophan (abundant in protein) to regulate serotonin. Depleted serotonin levels are a common factor of depression, and increasing levels have a proven positive effect. I have found that upping my protein intake with my own LynFit protein shakes

> **BUYING PROTEIN**
>
> WHETHER YOU use mine or another brand, you need high-quality whey per serving. Look for the following:
>
> 1) 20 to 25 grams of protein
> 2) 155 calories or fewer
> 3) Less than 1 gram of fat
> 4) Less than 15 grams of carbohydrates
> 5) No lactose, casein, or soy included

has truly made a difference in keeping my own depression at bay and allowing me to hear God's voice clearly.

The best way to get enough amino acids into your body is by taking a complete protein, which is a source of protein that includes all of the essential amino acids in the correct dietary proportion.

Three

THE LYNFIT DIFFERENCE

have spent my last 25 years researching and studying the science of supplementing. It is my passion and favorite thing to do every day—I am not happy if I am not learning something new. My quest began as a teenager as I always struggled with my weight and I took unnecessary risks when it came to weight loss drugs because I was so desperate. I too, was sold by advertising and TV personalities. I spent far too much of my hard-earned dollars buying countless bottles of supplements that I couldn't keep straight let alone take consistently everyday—not to mention it was too costly to keep up.

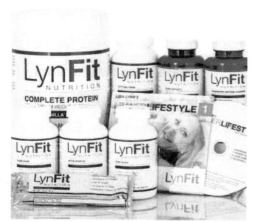

My passion became my purpose when I decided to create my own supplements. I dug deep into the science and asked biochemists why couldn't all the

> **THE LYNFIT LEAN PROMISE**
>
> I CARE MORE ABOUT YOU than my bottom line. I will be the "Brand with a Heart" that you can trust because I try everything myself first to guarantee that its 100 percent effective. If it isn't safe enough for my mom or kids, I won't sell it to you.

suggested nutrients be combined into one supplement? The answer had more to do with economics than science. By selling each supplement separately, companies had you buying 10 bottles instead of one and making much more money. In our current economy, eating healthy, eating cleanly, may not always be the most cost-effective to your wallet in the short-

> LynFit IS THE ABSOLUTE BEST OF MODERN SCIENCE IN FAT BURNING AND WEIGHT MANAGEMENT AND NOW THE EXPECTATION OF LIFELONG REAL RESULTS CAN BECOME A REALITY IF YOU FOLLOW *The Metabolism Solution* AS DIRECTED.

term (long-term results do make a difference) and buying and taking 10 or more different supplements that need to be taken consistently and frequently certainly isn't. This did not sit well with me. I took (and take) supplements daily because I know they help me, yet I am so frugal that I was having a hard time spending so much— even for my health. Yet I never questioned the amount of money spent on these products that were still keeping me fat. So I decided to make my own, all-in-one supplement.

Please note that certain nutrients like to be by themselves and work better that way, but others actually work better when they are synergistically and strategically combined with specific fellow nutrients. Think of a recipe: You wouldn't eat each ingredient on its own, but if you combine them per instruction, you get something tasty. When certain ingredients are

> WHEN CERTAIN INGREDIENTS ARE BLENDED TOGETHER, IT MAKES THEM 10 TIMES MORE EFFECTIVE.

blended together it makes them 10 times more effective.

Take raspberry ketones. I have used this supplement for over 25 years. There's nothing new about raspberry ketones. Fitness pros and models have used them for decades to lose the stubborn last 10 pounds or to force their bodies to burn that stubborn body fat that will not leave no matter how long they eat clean or how hard they exercise. Raspberry ketones like to be combined with other ingredients, specifically caffeine, which is one of the best fat burners of all time when used correctly. And since raspberry ketones are extremely expensive (four pounds of raspberries can go into making one capsule), caffeine makes certain that the nutrients are uploaded or taken up by the cells so they can be absorbed for better results and not just flushed out of the body. Why pay for a supplement that can't get to where it needs to go?

Martha Stewart was a great source of motivation and inspiration for me. When I was training Martha, who needed a metabolic push from supplements, I had to test every store-bought supplement for quality, purity, and ingredient accuracy before she took even one. The initial test results were shocking. The results came back with "unable to identify the ingredients." Not only were the store-bought supplements I provided to Martha expensive (Martha only buys the best), but their ingredients could not be identified. Store-brand supplements, generic supplements, may not be what they say they are. In fact, a 2013 Canadian study found that the labels of almost one-third of all supplements they examined did not match their contents. If you use these and don't see results, it could very well be that the quality of the supplements isn't high enough. Sadly I learned that many commercial brands are more interested in their profits than your results.

After the shock wore off from examining those unbelievable test results, I called my guru, Dr. Hatfield, and asked him about brands out there. I asked him if there was a supplement or shake out there that was high-quality and safe enough to give Martha Stewart. His reply was simple; "You need to make your own."

Just as Martha grows her own vegetables for freshness and quality assurance, I needed to make my own to know exactly what goes into them and be part of the entire process. I had no idea of what I was starting—no clue my life would be where it is today. Divine intervention.

> **LYNFIT ADVANTAGE**
> - **When you buy premium you'll need less.**
> - **With LynFit supplements you'll see results and feel better right away.**
> - **If you have old supplements laying around that you bought elsewhere and you don't see results within 2 weeks, you won't. So stop taking them. Throw them out.**

As I thought about Dr. Hatfield's advice to start my own supplement line, three realizations hit me: 1) People want to improve their health without hurting their bodies in the process; 2) They don't know what to take, how much to take, and when to take supplements.

The key to smart supplementing is to take exactly what your body needs—no more and no less—and timing is everything; and 3) Sluggish metabolisms need an extra push, and this is what I do best as I have one of the slowest metabolisms around.

SETTING THE STANDARD FOR EXCELLENCE

After watching Martha try to take her myriad of supplements daily—all those bottles, all those pills—supplements either from or endorsed by many world-renown experts—I decided to do my own research. Was there an easier way than taking so many different pills, capsules, and tablets? YES. The most important point I learned is that many of the supplements we need to take *can* be combined but are not because manufacturers want to make more profits. Everyone wants to make a profit, me too, but I am all about results. The only way to get results with supplements is to be consistent, to make them affordable so you can take them as long as needed and safe enough to take for the rest of your life. I set out to find the best manufacturers and scientists to create my own blends that would be highly effective and less expensive—and give results fast.

> WHEN I TOOK SUPPLEMENTS, I FELT BETTER. AND WHEN I FEEL BETTER, I EAT BETTER AND FEEL LIKE WORKING OUT. I CAN HEAR GOD'S VOICE LOUD AND CLEAR.

So my journey in supplement manufacturing began. I chose the top-quality ingredients and purchased them from the best suppliers, often checking with specialists on specific ingredients for advice. I called near every lab in the United States until I found someone who was excited about the prospect as I was.

Of course the first thing I wanted to know is if we could mix ingredients into one capsule. How many times did I ask; "If we know that taking B Complex, forskolin, suma root, white kidney bean extract, and other nutrients is the best way to enhance fat loss and kill cravings, why can't we blend them together into one capsule to be taken two times a day?"

For the best results, the right ingredients need to be combined so the body never adapts to only one ingredient and you always have a nutrient working for you all the time.

My research also taught me that the best way to take a supplement is in capsule form. A capsule delivers nutrients that are 30 percent more absorbable by the body. And a capsule can be emptied and poured into a liquid for optimal absorption. (That's what I do. I empty capsules right into my protein shake.)

I have taken the guesswork out of supplementing and made the LynFit brand to make it easy and affordable for you. I use only the highest quality nutrients, so you need to take less and will see results. Oh, you'll also feel better than you ever have in your life. My brand will never be sold in a store. Most times the quality goes down so profits can go up when supplements are sold in stores. I appreciate the efforts you go to order online and my LynFit *lean promise* to you is you will get the best results in the least amount of time—and you will never be sorry.

I have purchased more supplements out of desperation than I'd care to remember. If I could only have a dollar back for each bottle, I'd be rich. I want to spare you the pain, misery, and loss of your hard-earned dollars.

What makes LynFit different? It is backed by decades of scientific research and all of the products are made with premium ingredients, made right here in the United States in GMP-certified labs that are also FDA inspected. I love going to the plants and watching the process—I like to bless the mix.

SEVERAL SPECIFIC SUPPLEMENTS are extremely expensive and it's better to buy good quality than buy any at all. It's the What, Why, and How that's important.

I get the same questions every day: "What should I take to lose weight?" And my answer is always the same: "Take only what you need, when you need it." When you're living "clean" (eating right and exercising), you don't need to over-supplement.

You might be surprised to know that I am very conservative when it comes to supplements, and I believe in a keep-it-simple approach.

Supplements simply fill in the gaps your body might miss and assist your body in doing its job more effectively. God made your body in a spectacular-highly-intelligent-heal-thyself way, so living clean, eating right, and exercising is the best way to worship Him.

THE CUTTING EDGE

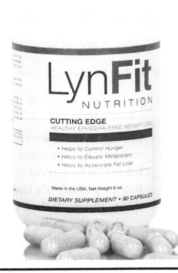

The first product I ever created was my Cutting Edge vitamin for weight loss. I loved this combination of ingredients for weight loss. I love the way it makes me feel and how I was able to lose those pounds right away. I used to purchase a similar blend from another company, but its quality slipped, so I made my own.

The ingredients in the Cutting Edge have been used for decades and modern research continues to validate them when it comes to losing stubborn body fat. L-Carnitine is the superstar in my Cutting Edge. It works as a shuttle, pulling fat from storage and dragging it into the cell so it can be burned off. And, combining L-Carnitine with 19 other highly effective fat-fighting agents who work together to fight fat from every angle means stubborn body fat doesn't stand a chance.

CUTTING EDGE

Suggested Usage: Take one (1) capsule three times a day with a full glass of water. For best results take a tablet at breakfast, another with lunch and a third at 3 p.m. (when your metabolism starts to slow).

LynFit Lean Tip: To really enhance your fat loss, try taking one to two Cutting Edge capsules right before a workout. It helps rev up your metabolism.

Supplementing with these nutrients is crucial. Without supplementation, we would need to eat an excess of fat in order to receive the dosage needed for fat loss, and that's counterproductive when it comes to losing body fat. With a Cutting Edge capsule, your body absorbs more of the nutrients than it would from food, especially since most foods high in these nutrients are also extremely high in fat. And mixing many of these nutrients with the B vitamins helps you metabolize them more efficiently.

> **CUTTING EDGE KEEPS FAT CELLS FROM GETTING BIGGER AND DECREASES BELLY FAT.**

All of the Essential Fatty Acids included in the Cutting Edge are good for every cell in the body: for cardiovascular health; lowering

> *"I lost more weight when I started taking Cutting Edge and I lost it without lots of exercise!"*   —L. T.

cholesterol levels; controlling diabetes; enhancing skin, nail, and hair health; for building up the immune system and for reducing all bodily inflammation, including inflammatory bowel disease. The Cutting Edge replaces lost nutrients that get depleted quickly when exercising and dieting and can improve sleep patterns, memory,

---

CUTTING EDGE COST COMPARISON

*Not only have I mixed the right nutrients
(in the right amounts) for you, but I'm made it cost-effective.**

LynFit Cutting Edge $38.95	vs.		
		Chromium Polynicotinate	$ 24.99
		L-Carnitine Complex	$ 34.99
		Choline Complex	$ 28.99
		Inositol	$ 13.49
		Vitamin B Complex	$ 14.99
		L-Methionine	$ 28.99
		Potassium Gluconate	$ 4.99
		Grapefruit Powder	$ 30.99
		Linolenic Acid	$ 20.49
		Chlorophyll	$ 14.99
			_____
			$217.90

*Pricing online supplements at time of publication.

and concentration while promoting HDL levels and lowering cholesterol levels. It's not a coincidence that many of the Cutting Edge's ingredients are used to treat Alzheimer's, liver ailments, and many, many more issues. The Cutting Edge helps stops fat cells from getting

> "I lost my belly fat taking 2 capsules of Cutting Edge daily—and I lowered my cholesterol!"   —A.Y.

bigger, and by decreasing abdominal fat, your weight loss is enhanced. It reduces blood sugar levels as well as cholesterol and triglyceride levels which helps increase your metabolic rate. This is especially important if you suffer from a slow thyroid. There isn't anyone who can't benefit from this supplement. It's in the Cutting Edge that I load you up with those superstar ingredients, specifically; L-Carnitine, Lecithin, Choline Complex, Inositol, and L-Menthionine.

COMPLETE PROTEIN

How do you get more protein and more of the *right* protein? Protein shakes. No, not those shakes you can buy in any convenience store as meal replacements, but sugar-free, high-grade, filler-free, lean protein. Models, celebrities, professional athletes all have one thing in common; they drink protein shakes as meal replacements. They all know how hard it is to lose weight and rid their bodies of excess body fat, and they know the value of a nutritious tool that makes their

> "Drinking Complete Protein shakes made losing 85 pounds easy. Living on the shake has helped me keep it off."   —J. R.

lives easier and is more cost-effective than focusing on specialty diet foods. What is this protein? Whey. Whey is a complete protein, containing all 20 amino acids and all 9 essential amino acids the body needs. It helps in muscle recovery and is widely considered to be the highest-quality natural protein.

Not all whey is created equal. The whey used in protein shakes favored by body builders who are looking to bulk up contains fat and lactose. Microfiltered, high-quality whey, which removes most of these two ingredients and is found in my own LynFit Complete

WHY DOES THE PER OF WHEY PROTEIN MAKE SUCH A BIG DIFFERENCE IN YOUR WEIGHT AND WAIST LOSS?

PER stands for Protein Efficiency Ratio, which, in basic terms, is a measure of how efficiently your body can use protein. Most of us who struggle to lose weight have sluggish digestive systems that aren't always the most efficient and don't break down proteins very well. Thus, proteins are more likely to get stored as fat since your body can't use them and they might upset your stomach and leave you feeling bloated. To avoid this, it's crucial to be aware of the PER of the food you eat and the shake you drink—especially when trying to lose weight. And high-quality whey is the #1 protein source when you want to boost your metabolism. Don't rely on an ad on television or in a magazine, read your labels.

Each protein is unique in its composition and how it affects your body. When it comes to protein shakes and bars, knowing the quality of protein and its source is of utmost importance if you're trying to lose weight and boost your metabolism. The simplest way to explain is that higher grades of whey are good for weight loss while less-expensive whey works well for bulking and adding weight as well as providing calories.

An acceptable PER score for a protein is 2.7. This is also known as a "standard" value. Notice it is a standard score; don't confuse it with a good value. Why quibble with semantics here? In order for a protein source to be good for weight loss it needs to be excellent, higher than 2.7. When it has an excellent PER then it can wear the label "Metabolic Boosting." Few products reach this rating, which is why you rarely see it on store shelves.

Technically speaking any protein that ranks above 2 is considered a good source of protein, only those that rank above 2.7 are considered an excellent source. Now this is a slippery slope: Just because a protein has an excellent PER does NOT mean it is good for weight loss. Take beef, for instance. It has a PER of 2.9, making it an excellent protein, but it is too high in fat to be good for your health and certainly won't help you burn fat. Casein, from milk sources, comes in at 2.7, also making it an excellent protein source, but it contains sugar, which is never a good thing when trying to boost a sluggish metabolism. Yogurt, full of casein, may be low-calorie but it won't help you lose weight. So why is whey the #1 protein source when it comes to PER while eggs actually have a higher score? Egg yolks are very high in fat; one yolk has 7 grams of fat, which is too much when trying to lose weight. Microfiltering whey makes it easier to digest and, thus, more efficiently used—even more than eggs—by your body.

RANKING PROTEINS BEST FOR WEIGHT LOSS BY PER	
1. Whey	3.2
2. Egg	3.9
3. Beef	2.9
4. Casein	2.7
5. Soy	2.2

The Secret to a Taste bud-Tantalizing, Metabolic-Boosting Protein Shake

Two scoops, a little water and ice, a shake, and you're good to go. But protein shakes made with LynFit Complete Protein powder can be so much more. The secret to boosting your metabolism using the protein shake lies in *how* you make one. Just remember, not all protein shakes are created equal. Use one like LynFit's Complete Protein that has 24 grams of high-quality, microfiltered whey that's low in calories, carbs, sugars, and fat. You never have to worry about quality using LynFit. After 25 years in the industry, I know how to make some fierce-tasting shakes that even the fussiest of palates will adore. Try these recipes or experiment on your own—but try to keep calorie-adding ingredients to a minimum if you want to get as much benefit out of protein as you can and still lose weight.

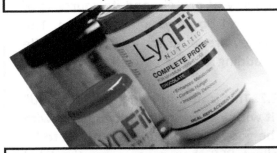

The Top 10 Best Ways to Use Complete Protein

1) Drink one immediately after a workout to nourish your muscles.
2) Add 1 tablespoon to your morning coffee instead of milk.
3) Try 1 to 2 scoops in your morning oatmeal.
4) Put Complete Protein in your favorite baked goods.
5) Add 1 tablespoon to yogurt or cottage cheese.
6) Enjoy as hot chocolate or light latte.
7) Sprinkle on top of fruit or dunk your fruit right into a pile of powder.
8) Add 1 tablespoon to your Jell-O mold.
9) Make popsicles by freezing already-made shakes.
10) Sprinkle on top of popcorn.

Blender Basics

1) Pour 1/2 cup cold water and begin mixing on lowest speed.
2) Add 2 scoops of your favorite flavor of LynFit Complete Protein powder and blend 10 seconds.
3) Gradually add 3 to 5 ice cubes (your preference) until completely blended.
4) Blend on high speed for 1 minute.

THICKER SHAKE?
Use less water and more ice.
CREAMIER SHAKE?
Blend longer at low speed.
NO BLENDER AND NO SHAKER CUP?
Add 1/4 cup water to Complete Protein powder and eat it like cake batter

Don't own a blender? That's OK, it's spoon-stirable.

MORE THAN A COMPLETE PROTEIN SHAKE

THE DETOXER
(AKA THE LEAN GREEN CLEANSING MACHINE)

Add 1 cup of your favorite baby greens to your vanilla shake while blending. Sweet, fresh, slightly tart. It hits all the spots.

BEAT THE BLOAT SMOOTHIE

Add 1 teaspoon of sugar-free banana Jell-O mix and 2 Cutting Edge to 2 scoops vanilla or chocolate Complete Protein to banish the bloat.

FUDGE FOR FASTER FAT LOSS
(AKA THE TRIPLE CHOCOLATE OVERLOAD)

Add 1 teaspoon sugar-free fudge pudding mix to 2 scoops chocolate Complete Protein to satisfy your chocolate craving.

PEANUT BUTTER AND CHOCOLATE
(AKA THE CRAVING KILLER)

Add 1 teaspoon of PB2 peanut butter powder to 2 scoops of chocolate Complete Protein to stop the noshing.

RASPBERRY KETONE FAT SHREDDER
(AKA MIRACLE IN A BLENDER)

Empty 1 Accelerator capsule into 2 scoops of chocolate Complete Protein to rev up your metabolism even more.

FIBERIZER
(AKA THE BOWEL BOMB)

Add 1 level scoop of Sunfiber to your favorite flavor for regularity.

Try a shake warm as a "skinny hot chocolate"

RESEARCHERS AT SYRACUSE UNIVERSITY FOUND THAT:

- **Drinking a clean protein shake before your work out speeds fat loss.**
- **People who drank a clean, low-carb whey protein shake daily had higher metabolic rates.**
- **Drinking a clean whey protein shake that provided adequate protein helped to lower the stress hormone cortisol, boosting metabolism.**
- **Overeating dampens your dopamine response while drinking a shake combats this.**

LEAN OUT LEMON

Add 1 to 2 teaspoons sugar-free lemon Jell-O mix to 2 scoops vanilla Complete Protein when you need something tart.

CINNAMON VANILLA DECADENCE

Warm or cold, add 1 teaspoon cinnamon to your vanilla Complete Protein to help lower blood sugar.

ORANGE-VANILLALICIOUS

Add 1 teaspoon sugar-free orange Jell-O to 2 scoops vanilla Complete Protein for a great carb-free drink.

METABOLIC MOCHACCINO
(AKA THE ENERGIZER)

Add 1 to 1 1/2 teaspoon granulated coffee to 2 scoops vanilla or chocolate Complete Protein for a fat-melting pick-me-up.

Protein is the fat-busting protein of choice. I use whey concentrate in my protein powder. Whey is typically processed into three forms; powder, concentrate and isolate. Whey powder is one of the most common additives in the food industry, used from meat products to baked

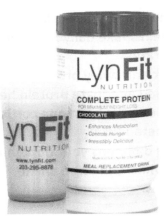

goods. To make whey concentrate, the whey is processed to remove water, lactose, ash, and minerals, filtering it for optimum health benefit. To create whey isolate, whey concentrate is processed even further, breaking down some of the substances that make whey beneficial for weight loss while allowing other beneficial substances to enter your bloodstream faster and go to work quicker. Whey concentrate is most popular in protein shakes.

Taste is another indicator of whey grade. Pure whey tastes terrible. It has to be sweetened to be made palatable. Although we all hate to see sugar, sweeteners, or any carbs on the label (The amount of sweetener in my own LynFit brand of whey protein is so minimal

> **COMPLETE PROTEIN**
> **Suggested Usage:** Use 2 level scoops with 1 cup of cold water for a delicious meal-replacement shake or as an afternoon snack
> **LynFit Lean Tip:** Make one day a week a Shake Day, drinking shakes for your meals, to breakthrough weight loss plateaus and burn off stubborn fat.

it is barely measurable and doesn't need to be on the label by law. But I choose to let you know exactly what is in my whey.), it is important to keep perspective and understand that some carbs are *necessary*. Do not fall into the trap of thinking that if low-carb is good than no-carb must be better. Nutrition is a science. We need a small

amount of specific carbohydrates to guarantee that protein gets transported into our cells in order for them to be used and not stored as fat. LynFit's Complete Protein is one of the lowest in carbs and sugar on the market but it tastes the best. Even Martha Stewart thinks so—after all she was my tester when I was creating these shakes. I use only natural flavorings; chocolate, vanilla, and strawberry.

Flavor is key. If it tastes good, you'll drink it. And the more shakes you drink the more weight you will lose. It's that simple. Drinking shakes helps you move away from the foods that trigger cravings and cause your insulin to spike, making you gain that tire around your middle. A shake for breakfast—and if you want to burn fat faster substitute a shake for lunch—will help you reach your goal. A 3pm shake can be that perfect pick-me-up that stops you from reaching for that bag of chips or overloading on dinner.

> *"I lost two pounds a day since I started drinking the Complete Protein shake. Nothing was working before."* —E.B.

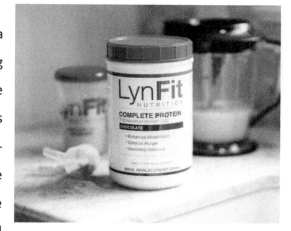

You will not see the same results using a lower-grade whey product. In fact, if you are using protein shakes for meal replacements and don't see results within two weeks and don't feel cravings dissipating, then you are using cheap whey. High-grade whey like that used in LynFit's Complete Protein is geared toward fat and weight loss while many other commercial brands are geared toward adding muscle bulk and weight gain. And many of these products contain so much sugar and other fillers like soy that they are no healthier than a high-calorie dessert.

How do you know if your whey is from a high-grade source and microfiltered? As you might expect, price is an indicator. If you buy cheap whey, you get cheap whey. At press time, a pound of high-quality whey runs about $25 a pound and is *never mixed* with vitamins, dairy, soy, milk products, gluten, or any wannabe-whey proteins such as pea or potato protein.

Through research and years of studying effects on myself and my clients, I have found a few magic ingredients that can change your life. I've spoken about them on Dr. Oz and other television and radio shows and received tons of questions about them. That's one of the reasons that prompted me to write this book. Supplements can be the ultimate quick fix when used in conjunction with a thermogenic diet and metabolic exercise.

THE TOP TEN SUPPLEMENTS TO BLAST FAT AND BOOST YOUR METABOLISM

1) **COMPLETE PROTEIN SHAKE** Boosts metabolism 25 percent while building metabolism so it's ready to be boosted.

2) **LEAN BARS** Boosts metabolism 25 percent, builds metabolism and provides prebiotics to boost immunity and fiber to fill you up. Satisfies the need to chew.

3) **CARB EDGE** Blocks 65 percent of unwanted carbs and fat while killing cravings and enhancing the metabolism.

4) **CUTTING EDGE** Encourages your body to burn fat while B complex enhances calorie burn and helps ease muscle soreness.

5) **PURE OMEGA-3** Balances blood sugar, improves fat burning, and boosts immunity.

6) **ACCELERATOR** Slices up fat cells making them easier to burn and affects adiponectin levels tricking your bodies into thinking like a thin person. Boosts you through plateaus.

7) **LEAN SLEEP** Burns fat while you sleep, and sleep is a critical component of the weigh-loss process. Helps you sleep better and lean.

8) **RASPBERRY KETONE CLEANSE** Helps detox your body and makes fat burning easier.

9) **DAILY POWER SHOT** Energizes and nourishes.

10) **RECOVERY AGENT** Helps with aches and pains that can stop weight loss in its tracks by slowing your metabolism.

CARB EDGE

The No. 1 rated TV health show in the United States, *The Dr. Oz Show*, has featured white kidney bean extract, forskolin, guggulsterone, and banaba leaf extract in weight loss segments. The shows' producers were very impressed by them and how these supplements may help in the weight loss struggle. I'm impressed by them, too, and have used them for years.

There are many obstacles on the path to weight loss. A sluggish metabolism, low thyroid function, insatiable cravings, and lack of energy are only the tip of the iceberg. These issues stop us from doing what we need to do to reach our weight loss and fitness goals. When they pop up we lack motivation to make better choices—and that's why they need to be addressed. I believe God has provided us with everything we need to overcome these obstacles and I put all that good stuff in my Carb Edge. You can overcome your fat battle for good without any of the harmful side effects that weight loss medications or surgical treatments bring. And you don't need to spend outrageous amounts of money to only be left more depressed and heavier than ever. I personally hate taking medications (of course I do, when absolutely necessary), and living following *The Metabolism Solution* brings me relief from an under-performing thyroid, cravings, lack of energy, and even mild depression.

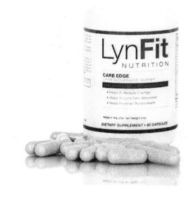

CARB EDGE
Suggested Usage: Take one (1) capsule two to three times a day with meals.
LynFit Lean Tip: Take Carb Edge 30 minutes before a "cheat" meal to block 65 percent of the unwanted carbs from being digested.

Since television only provides two to three minutes of explanation, I want to give you more. I want to take the time to explain what's in my Carb Edge (and all my products) and how it may benefit you. I want you to make informed choices and not be led by fads or extreme claims.

> *"Carb cravings were becoming unmanageable until I started taking Carb Edge every day."* —A.H.

I carefully put together the nutrients in Carb Edge—one safe supplement to save you time and money and help you lose weight. I keep coming back to many of those superstar ingredients discussed in the previous chapter. They make a winning combination when it comes to the battle of the bulge.

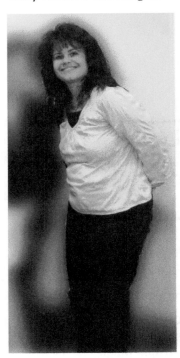 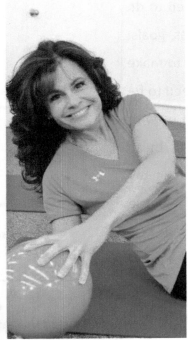

Dana – Lost 34 Pounds And Got In Shape!

Real People. Real Results.
While all people are different and individual results will vary, these photos are of LynFit's customers' actual experience.

Carb Edge is best known for its revolutionary new metabolic-boosting properties. It contains not one, not two, but *seven* different superstar fat busters that can help get the weight off.

White kidney bean extract, specifically Phase 2, is for you if you crave carbs and can't stop. White kidney bean extract blocks up to 65 percent of unwanted carbs from being absorbed. All that sugar isn't stored and turned into fat and your blood sugar levels are more level so you may be less likely to eat more. (Who wants to get caught in the vicious cycle of binging, feeling guilty, and then eating more?) If you take a Carb Edge at Noon and again at 3pm, you may find you crave less, and when food is placed in front of you, you're less likely to indulge. Taking a diet day off? Take a Carb Edge 30 minutes before your cheat meal and you may block carbs from being absorbed. If they're blocked, you'll never have to burn them off.

Forskolin is a metabolism enhancer and I specifically chose to add it to my Carb Edge supplement because this safe and highly effective ingredient helps wake up a sleeping metabolism. It helps to protect and build lean muscles tissue so you can continue to burn more calories even at rest.

Forskolin also aids in the production of thyroid hormone and promotes its release so it helps to keep your thyroid regulated while losing weight. When you restrict calories in your diet your thyroid slows down your metabolism, leaving your body wanting to conserve as much energy as possible. And that's the irony. You need to eat less to lose weight—it's the only proven method that works—but once you restrict your calories your metabolism may work against weight loss. Forskolin is crucial for lasting weight loss and in ensuring your thyroid works optimally.

> *"I dropped four clothes sizes and my stomach is now flat with Carb Edge."*
>
> —C. L.

Guggul (guggolsterone) another superstar, is best known for keeping all physiological fat burning systems operating at a maximum capacity by increasing your metabolic rate. It is effective even on low-calorie diets, so you can change your body dramatically since you're burning stubborn body fat. It may help you lose weight faster and easier without ever slowing down your thyroid. Like forskolin, guggul works best when combined with other fat-burning, metabolic-boosting ingredients. Instead of just one workhorse, you have five or more ingredients working to help you lose weight and fat.

Banaba Leaf is included in Carb Edge because it is a plant whose leaves are high in plant insulin known as corsolic acid. Banaba Leaf has been used for antidiabetic purposes in

Ayurvedic medicine as well as in other cultures for over 2,000 years to help lower and regulate blood sugar levels. In my opinion, Banaba leaf extract is one the very best blood sugar lowering supplements on the market.

I've seen blood sugar levels lowered using banaba leaf that couldn't be lowered with exercise and diet. Lowering blood sugar is the first priority when trying to get your body to shed fat, so adding banaba leaf to my Carb Edge was a no brainier. Not to mention it helps control cravings as most of them start out as blood sugar issues. Lower the blood sugar and anybody can burn fat.

Alpha lipoic acid, also known as thiotic acid, is a naturally occurring compound, a powerful antioxidant that is made by the body in small amounts and is found in every cell. Its main function is to helps turn glucose into energy, lowering blood sugar levels. It is both fat- and water-soluable and therefore can work on every part of the body. Alpha lipoic acid works with B vitamins to produce energy from proteins, carbohydrates, and fats consumed through foods. It is best known for its help with metabolic syndrome and is used for diabetes. Recent studies have shown that alpha lipoic acid may affect thyroid hormones.

> **BLACK TEA VS. GREEN TEA GREEN TEA IS HIGH IN POLYPHENOLS. RESEARCHERS NOW THINK BLACK TEA MAY BE JUST AS GOOD FOR YOU.**

Suma root extract and black tea round out the superstars in Carb Edge. Suma root, known as Brazilian ginseng (although it is not related to ginseng), comes from the suma vine grown in South America that has been used in traditional herbal medicine for centuries. It helps to boost the immune system, helping the body deal with stress and balancing blood sugar levels. Russian scientific studies have shown that suma root increases lean muscle while reducing body fat.

Black tea comes from the same plant as green tea. It turns black because the leaves are thoroughly oxidized—exposed to oxygen. Black tea and green tea differ in how they are processed, which controls how many polyphenols (antioxidants that may help in weight loss) are in the tea. A study in Japan published in a March 2011 issue of *Nutrition* showed that mice fed black tea extract lost weight and reduced the amount of fat in their livers. Researchers at Poland's University of Warsaw published another study in the *European Journal of Nutrition* (also in March 2011) finding that supplementing with black tea, because of its flavonoids, could reduce blood glucose. Black tea may very well help boost your metabolism.

THE LEAN BAR

Who says you won't crave food that's good for you? Getting Lean is all about feeding the muscle and starving the fat into leaving. And that's what makes my Lean Bars so unique. They are the only protein bar on the market specifically designed for weight loss. Unlike other brands out there (and I've tried them all), only Lean Bars are made with a premium-grade whey protein (remember, studies have shown it can temporarily boost your calorie burn) as well as 10 grams of filling prebiotic inulin fiber, a

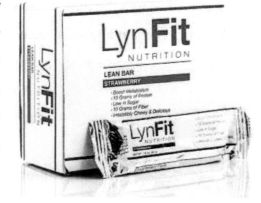

natural, dietary fiber (the same healthy fiber found in fruits and vegetables) that helps support your immune system and your digestive tract.

> **LEAN BAR**
> **Suggested Usage:** Enjoy one to two Lean Bars per day as a snack or meal replacement.
> **LynFit Lean Tip:** Can't stop cravings? Replace your trigger food with a Lean Bar instead. They come in five delicious flavors: strawberry, chocolate, peanut butter, toffee, and Tahitian vanilla. Have a Lean Bar anytime you'd have a Complete Protein shake.

You've probably heard more about probiotics than prebiotics thanks to all those yogurt commercials on television. But don't confuse the two. Prebiotics are not probiotics. Probiotics are live organisms, good bacteria that help keep your digestive tract operating smoothly (pun intended) and your immune system at optimum strength. They are sensitive to heat and light and can be killed by stomach acid—before they are even digested. Prebiotics are, in essence, food for the probiotics. They are not organisms but mostly carbohydrates (fiber) that the human body cannot digest.

> *"Delicious, satisfying, healthy perfect for a meal on- the-go or to add to my children's lunch box for an after school snack or for recovery from sports events. I think my family is going to snack themselves to six pack."*   —V.S.

What makes prebiotics especially interesting is a recent study published in the journal *Science* in September of 2013. Researchers found a correlation between gut bacteria and obesity. Using mice, they took fecal bacteria from sets of twins, one lean, and one heavy. Mice given the bacteria from the lean twins lost weight. Mice getting gut bacteria from the heavier twins, gained. When the now obese mice were given bacteria from the leaner twins, they then lost weight. The already lean mice never gained weight when given bacteria from heavier donors. From this and other studies, researchers are convinced that your gut bacteria has an effect on how well you burn and store fat. And I agree with them.

LEAN BARS HAVE AS MUCH FIBER AS 4 CUPS OF BROCCOLI AND AS MUCH PROTEIN AS 3 OZ. OF CHICKEN—WITHOUT ALL THE FAT AND CALORIES. THEY FEED MUSCLE AND STARVE FAT—PERFECT FOR WEIGHT LOSS.

A different study showed that a mere 8 grams of prebiotic inulin fiber can help ease pain, bloating and constipation associated with irritable bowels and help keep you regular which is key when you're trying to lose weight. Animal studies have even indicated that prebiotics may protect against early stage colon cancer. While others propose they lower triglycerides and control blood sugar levels.

The LynFit Lean Bar comes in five outrageously delicious flavors that satisfy your cravings and keep you feeling full. It took many months of research to create a line of lean bars that satisfy that craving. I crave foods as much as the next person; cravings don't go away. It's all about replacing the fattening stuff with a healthier, lean version. These are the top five flavors, as my many clients suggested.

1) Chewy Chocolate. Who can resist chocolate? Definitely not me. The chocolate lean bar is one chocolate that's good for weight loss. And the fact that it tastes like a Tootsie Roll doesn't hurt.
2) Peanut Butter. A blissfully delicious flavor that keeps you out of the peanut butter jar. And it tastes like you just grabbed a spoonful straight from your favorite brand. A kid's favorite lunch box snack.
3) Tahitian Vanilla. The vanilla connoisseur will find nirvana here. No bland vanilla here, but pure taste that's delightfully delicious and filling.
4) Toffee. A classic favorite for just about everyone. We all deserve a treat.
5) Strawberry. For the fruit lover, a divinely delicious and refreshing treat.

> **LEAN BAR BENEFITS**
> 1) 20 grams of high-quality whey protein
> 2) 2.5 grams of sugar
> 3) 10 grams of fiber
> 4) 11 net carbs; soy- and gluten-free

How much do you spend on snacks for your family and yourself? Did you know that the average junk food purchase in the United States is $3.75 at one time? Think about it; $3.75 for junk food that will make you gain weight, or $2.91 for a filling, good-for-you protein bar? No contest.

Another thing to keep in mind: If you're paying less than $2.75 for a protein bar, you're not getting premium whey or the right nutrients to help your body lose weight. Just about every protein bar on the market is made with inferior ingredients like soy, gluten, and

THE BEST TIME FOR A LEAN BAR IS… ANYTIME

➢ Have a Lean Bar to replace a meal or as a snack when trying to lose weight and body fat. Eat one anytime to replace a protein shake.
➢ After a workout. This is the time your body is screaming for nutrients like protein.
➢ Not trying to lose weight and just want to be healthy? No problem. Simply add a lean bar to your day whenever you feel the urge to snack—especially after working out or activity.
➢ While traveling. Never leave home without extra Lean Bars. They are great for the airport, car rides, and lunch boxes.

sugar—the perfect food for gaining weight. But if weight loss is your goal you need the right nutrients to fuel your metabolism. That's what separates the lean bar from every single other bar on the market.

> "I feel like I'm cheating on my diet. LynFIT thank you for creating a healthy, all-natural scrumptious snack. Peanut Butter is my favorite for those moments when I crave peanut butter but don't want to break my diet."   —J. G

Lean Bars are the only bar on the market that will help you lose weight and boost your metabolism. You also burn fat while feeding your lean muscle so it stays tight and firm. If you replace your current snack with Lean Bar, you can lose weight faster and easier.

But I should warn you that Lean Bars are addicting. Once you try a Lean Bar you will never live without them.

ACCELERATOR

This was my first raspberry ketone product. I have supplemented with raspberry ketones for over 25 years. My LynFit Accelerator has five key ingredients that work together with raspberry ketones:

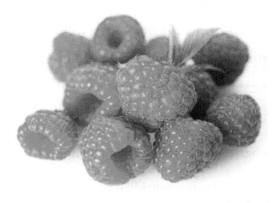

1) B6 and B12 vitamins to help assimilate and break down ingredients so that they are better utilized and to help guarantee that your food is always broken down and used for energy
2) Green Tea Leaf Extract for better absorption
3) Chromium to lower blood sugar so you lose fat faster and easier
4) Chocolate Bean Powder to make you feel better and increase fat loss
5) Caffeine, as much as you'd find in a small cup of coffee to guarantee nutrient uptake.

My Accelerator is a unique blend of nutrients designed to boost the fat-burning process.

Mixing all these together is far more effective than taking them individually (and cheaper). This special

> *"I couldn't lose the fat until I took the Accelerator."*   —S.D.

blend of herbs and nutrients acts as a catalyst to jumpstart your metabolism and create a feeling of fullness to enhance the fat-burning process. These ingredients may help rid your body of excess water, balance blood sugar levels, and generate energy so you can exercise easier.

The raspberry ketones I use in my product are grown in the United States. They are the red-fruited raspberries typically grown in North America that stem from *Rubus idaeus*, scientifically, and its horticultural derivative *Rubus strigosus*. Some supplement companies use all parts of the plant, I use the fruit itself, the most effective part. The fruit contains folic acid and vitamin C that help provide antioxidant protection. It's the compound found in the fruit that works the "miracles".

I've combined the most effective ingredients for fat loss in this product and that's what makes my product different. Raspberry ketones are great, but combined with green tea leaf extract and chocolate bean powder, you always have at least two superstar fat fighters working instead of one. The combination of raspberry ketones, green tea leaf extract, chocolate bean powder, vitamins B6 and B12, and chromium can decrease visceral fat by 12 percent more than when taking raspberry ketones alone, reducing your waist size in a matter of weeks.

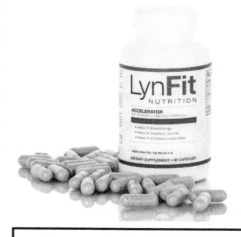

ACCELERATOR
Suggested Usage: Take (1) capsule first thing in the morning and another if needed at lunch time.
LynFit Lean Tip: Take an Accelerator before you work out to accelerate your fat loss and bust through plateaus.

Green Tea is one of the best ways to guarantee that raspberry ketones are absorbed and work fast. This is also why supplementing is the way to get the best results—you would have to eat far too many pounds of raspberries to get the same amount of ketones found in one capsule. Even if you were able to eat pounds of raspberries a day, you would not get the same results. Why? Without the added green tea, raspberry ketones don't absorb well into the body. This super combo allows the Accelerator to work faster in the body decreasing the absorption time and increasing its effectiveness.

The recommended dosage is one capsule first thing in the morning and another, if needed, (when you're having a bad eating day) at lunchtime. You never need to take more

> *"I broke through a plateau and lost those last stubborn pounds with the Accelerator."*   —C.T.

than two a day and it is better taken before 3pm if you are a light sleeper. If you are prone to anxiety or have high blood pressure, you should use caution in taking the Accelerator until your blood pressure is under control or you are feeling less anxious. Instead, you can take my Raspberry Ketone Cleanse (see page 75), which contains the same high-quality raspberry ketones and is blended with a caffeine-free combination, as an alternative.

The Accelerator is a great way to break through weight loss plateaus and ramp up your metabolism after some bad eating days. If you are replacing two meals a day with a LynFit Complete Protein Shake or Lean Bar and your diet is clean enough (80 percent of the time) but your weight remains stuck, add the Accelerator to your daily supplements to bust out of the plateau. And remember; you cannot supplement or exercise away a bad diet.

PURE OMEGA-3

Omega fatty acids are the only Fat that helps burn fat. If I had to choose among my supplements, this is the one that everyone should take daily. Every person in my home takes

Pure Omega-3 every day—I even give it to my dogs. Pure Omega-3 also supports healthy heart and cardiovascular function, healthy joints and

> "Taking LynFit's Pure Omega-3 helped me lose 15 pounds and cleaned up my skin too."
> —D. M.

normal flexibility, brain health and normal focus and mood, and healthy skin and circulation. If you've stayed with me this far, you know what I say; if you don't see results in two weeks stop taking the supplement, you most likely won't. Often, you won't see results because the quality of the supplement isn't high enough, it doesn't use high-quality, premium ingredients. This holds especially true for Omega-3 supplements.

Most store brands of fish oil contain only 5 to 25 percent Omega-3 fatty acids and the rest comes from saturated fats, Omega-6's. Yep, the fats that cause weight gain. Most Americans consume enough Omega-6 fatty acids that the recommended dosage on the bottle would be too low in keeping your Omega-3 to Omega-6 ratio in check, which is one of the primary goals of supplementing fish oil. In fact, Americans eat up to 10 times more Omega-6's than Omega-3's. Some brands may seem inexpensive, but that's because they don't go through the process of removing impurities like mercury. And many brands include Omega-3 from chia or flax, which has been shown to be not as effective as Omega-3's from fish; plant sources just don't measure up.

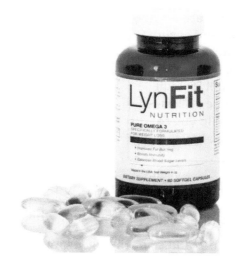

PURE OMEGA 3
Suggested Usage: Take 2 soft gel tablets daily with a meal or as directed by your healthcare professional.
LynFit Lean Tip: Are you hungrier in the afternoon than during other parts of the day? Take one Pure Omega-3 at 3 p.m. to help conquer your cravings.

Did you know that Omega-3 from a fish source is the most effective at helping your body to burn fat by lowering and or balancing your blood sugar levels and that other supplements used to provide Omega-3 such as flax, chia, or anything that doesn't say Omega-3 from fish can actually be stopping your weight loss? LynFit's Pure Omega-3 contains the exact combination of EPA & DHA that your body needs to help with: insatiable cravings, improving fat burning, balancing blood sugar levels, boosting immune function, helping to maintain healthy triglycerides. In addition, Pure Omega-3 may reduce the risk of coronary artery disease, help ease depression, help with brain cognitive function and joint mobility, and even help in making hair and skin healthy.

CURB CRAVINGS

Taking Pure Omega-3 at 3 p.m. is a trick I use to help fight off cravings. Good fats take longer to digest, so if you take Pure Omega-3 in the morning with your Complete Protein shake and again around 3 p.m. before that crazy craving time we all deal with, you'll feel full when meal time strikes— and this will help you to eat smaller meals.

LynFit's Pure Omega-3 is 80 percent pure fish oil. That's the highest and purest you can get. It's pure and free of all impurities. Hence, the "Pure" in the name. You'll find no Omega-6's in my brand as I will not include a pro-inflammatory that *counteracts* Omega-3 when trying to lose weight. And the best added plus with Pure Omega-3; no fish burps. It's so fresh you can chew it. If it were any fresher it would be moving. My premium grade Pure Omega-3 is the same strength as prescription-strength Omega-3 available in Europe, which is used to treat just about every ailment and promote health. I add a purifying proprietary antioxidant blend of rosemary extract and natural tocotrienols to retain its freshness and prevent oxidation as well as a delicious lemon flavor.

"I lost my belly fat and I'm not achy anymore. Two Pure Omega 3s a day— that's all it took.   —J.R.

With LynFit's Pure Omega-3 you can be sure that you are getting a pharmaceutical-grade, super-concentrated fish oil that contains exactly the amount of EPA and DHA your body needs: 1500 mg of Omega 3 per serving. That's 800 mg from EPA and 600 mg from DHA and no fishy after taste. And it's three times the amount of Omega-3's than regular fish oil supplements. I suggest taking 1 Pure Omega-3 capsule at lunch time and another again at 3pm—right before the munchies set in—to help curb cravings.

Keep forgetting to take your Pure Omega-3? Then try taking two when you get up instead. It's better to be consistent. While my Pure Omega-3 capsules are smaller than others out there, they still pack a punch. And if swallowing is an issue, you can always open your Pure Omega 3 capsule (or any one of my capsules) and put it in food (or in a Complete Protein Shake).

RECOVERY AGENT

If you have one of those achy bodies or maybe your workouts make you sore, working out too hard or aggravating old injuries can send you reaching for pain relief. And if you suffer from joint discomfort, you've probably tried a variety of supplements. Tedious gels, pills, powders, and creams. How well do they really work? It seems every year joint companies tout the next big thing; their latest products are "revolutionary", "ground-breaking" and "shocking". But what has actually changed? Your pain may very well remain—as well as those extra pounds.

> PAIN MEDS CAN STOP THE HEALING PROCESS AND SLOW METABOLISM.

The worst part is that many of these pain medications and supplements can negatively affect your metabolism (aka: slow it down) and thus make weight loss impossible. That's why I created Recovery Agent. We all suffer with sore, painful joints at one time or another—whether it be from overuse, injury, arthritis, bursitis tendonitis, or maybe even healing from surgery or an illness. Whatever the cause, your body needs additional nutritional support to heal and repair from the inside out. When our bodies are sick or under stress, our nutrient needs are increased and diet alone is almost never enough. That's where Recovery Agent comes in. Recovery Agent is a combination of 16 of the highest-quality ingredients in exactly the amount your body needs to be effective. Researchers have discovered that when certain nutrients are combined in a concentrated form they are more powerful. Recovery Agent is a multivitamin and pain/joint protector wrapped up into one. We all need to prevent injuries and joint pain from happening in the first place, so why not provide your body with the nutrients that keep your joints supple and pliable and replace the nutrients lost when exercising or from age-related decline as well as over-use injuries?

> *"I took Recovery Agent when I was healing from hip surgery. I healed so fast the doctor wanted to know what I was taking. "* —M.V.

Recovery Agent is a powerful yet safe and effective supplement for both men and women. It utilizes the body's multiple pathways and systems to promote aggressive healing and recovery to fight off inflammation that causes pain. Arthritis, tendonitis, bursitis, or any "itis" for that matter may be relieved taking LynFit's Recovery Agent without hurting or slowing your metabolism.

It's all about the healing, and when our bodies heal, inflammation is reduced and pain goes away. Why cover the pain issue with harmful medications that can actually delay healing and some may even stop the healing process? With Recovery Agent you can heal at the source of the injury and your joints and body will feel better than ever.

Recovery and repair of tissues requires a host of vitamins and minerals that participate in the process, and Recovery Agent is a unique blend of exactly the right combination of vitamins, minerals, and antioxidants that have an anti-inflammatory effect and speed the rate of tissue repair and healing.

You'll find these in Recovery Agent:

- Vitamin A for boosting your body's immune function/response

- Vitamin C to protect your cells from radical damage and support connective tissue and prevent joint deterioration
- Vitamin E, an antioxidant that helps support your brain and carries tremendous benefits for joint protection, reducing joint destruction, and great for healing and repair
- Zinc to reduce pain and inflammation by helping calcium be absorbed more efficiently by your bones
- Glucosamine sulfate, an amino sugar that plays a crucial role in the formation of joint cartilage

Perhaps most important of all is L-Glutamine. This kingpin of amino acids is a superstar ingredient in Recovery Agent and known to be one of the best healing nutrients available. L-Glutamine provides additional nutritional support when your body is healing or recovering from illness, workouts, stress, surgery, or a chronic condition. It is known to play a role in keeping your muscle cells, immune system, and digestive system healthy. I put it in my LynFit brand because L-Glutamine is also known to diminish sugar and alcohol cravings. Why is this important? When you consume too much sugar it causes excess inflammation and you feel more pain. By eating less sugar, your inflammation decreases and your cravings diminish if not disappear.

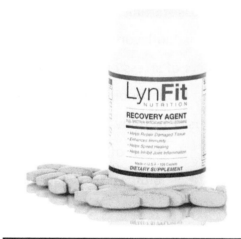

RECOVERY AGENT
Suggested Usage: Dosage varies with weight and activity levels. See product label. Recommended for anyone who is on a weight loss or fitness program, under stress, or interested in adding key nutrients related to improving heart health.
LynFit Lean Tip: Take immediately before and after your workout/activity for best healing.

Also worth talking about is curcumin, another ingredient in Recovery Agent. It is an antioxidant and an ingredient in the spice turmeric. According to the American Cancer

Society, turmeric is being tested to see if it can slow the growth of cancer cells in humans as it has done so in a laboratory. Turmeric, as well as its active ingredient curcumin, is an anti-inflammatory that many claim has fewer side effects than typical over-the-counter pain relievers. Most often used to flavor and color Asian cooking, curcumin is five to eight times stronger than vitamin E and vitamin C and may help boost your immune system, maintain normal cholesterol levels, and put the brakes on aging. It has even been considered in treatment for Alzheimer's patients as a way to slow down the brain inflammation associated with the disease. The icing on the cake with curcumin is that it is thermogenic—it naturally boosts your metabolism to help you burn calories. (See Chapter 4, Thermogenic Eating for Radical Weight Loss starting on page 85 for more)

I put Citrus bioflavonoids in Recovery Agent because they provide a strong defense against the effects of stress on the body. They are perfect for weight loss because they also inhibit bone loss. Bioflavonoids, also known as flavonoids, are derived from plants and most common in citrus. Our body takes in most bioflavonoids from our diets, but also excretes most of it because it is so easily processed. Preliminary research shows bioflavonoids have promise for allergies and inflammation.

L-GLUTAMINE DIMINISHES ALCOHOL AND SUGAR CRAVINGS.

Green tea extract is one of those ingredients you hear touted all the time for weight loss. It may decreases appetite while increasing your metabolism. But did you know that alongside glucosamine and chondroitin, it is also good for joints? Dr. Oz even recommends it. Green tea is high in EGCG (epigallocatechin gallate, a very potent antioxidant) and ECG (epicatechin gallate, a flavonoid). These two ingredients have been shown to regulate and inhibit cancer growth in some studies, especially for those with prostate and breast cancers, as well as help against inflammation. Bromelain (also known as Bromelin) is an enzyme found in pineapple juice and in the pineapple stem and in Recovery Agent. It has been long used in folk and alternative medicine in Central and South America. It is helpful in reducing swelling and pain. And of special note, Bromelain is believed to help the body get rid of excess fat. It is commonly found in common meat tenderizers as it helps break protein down and, thus, "softens" the meat.

> "I was having trouble with pain from back surgery and was taking lots of medications that caused me to gain weight and slowed my metabolism. Then I started taking Recovery Agent twice a day and now I feel better than I have in years."   —D.J.

The Siberian ginseng (also known as eleuthero) found in Recovery Agent also helps with pain and swelling and can help increase physical stamina and the ability to handle stress. It has long been used in traditional Chinese medicine and comes from the roots of a shrub that grows in Russia, China, Korea, and Japan. Part of the ginseng family, long known for its beneficial properties, Siberian ginseng can help strengthen the immune system.

Bilberry extract is in Recovery Agent because it too is a powerful antioxidant and anti-inflammatory—and it's great for leg cramps. Bilberries are related to that known high-powered antioxidant the blueberry and are indigenous to Northern Europe. They are an excellent source of flavonoids and have been shown to help with various eye ailments. A study using mice in Japan also noted that bilberries may be beneficial in reducing the risk of diabetes. Further studies are being conducted.

> RECOVERY AGENT IS YOUR MAGIC BULLET FOR PAIN RELIEF AND FAT LOSS. CLEAN OUT YOUR LIVER-CLOGGING MEDICINE CABINET.

Ginkgo biloba can help reduce joint pain, so of course I put it in Recovery Agent. Long thought to help with memory issues and blood flow problems, ginkgo biloba may also lessen inflammation and provide antioxidant support in fighting cell damage.

Capsicum has also been long-used to relieve pain, improve circulation, treat cluster headaches and psoriasis, and even help with weight loss. You may know it better as the chile pepper—cayenne, an important spice used around the world. Hot red peppers that produce capsicum are a thermogenic food. You need to burn more calories to digest it than are found

> *"My rheumatologist cannot believe that by losing weight and taking Recovery Agent I am off ALL meds."*   -DN

in the pepper itself. A study in the Netherlands in 2005 showed that people given capsicum with meals had increased satiety and calorie burning with suppressed appetite. Did you know that Recovery Agent may also keep you satiated and suppress your appetite? Ongoing clinical trials hope to build on the University of Maryland Medical Center reports that show that capsicum supplements may increase a body's heat production for a brief period and regulate blood sugar levels by their effect on the breakdown of carbohydrates during digestion.

Because of the caffeine contained within, the Kola nut (yes, the one that brings the flavor to all colas and makes you feel good) can help with drowsiness and fatigue. Since it is not addictive and does not lead to depression, the *Journal of the American Medical Association* recommends using the Kola nut over other stimulants. Used for healing and flavoring for centuries in Africa where it originally grew but now can be found in Brazil and

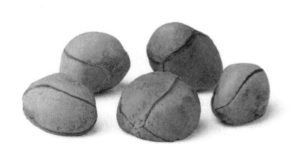

the Caribbean as well, it also acts as an appetite suppressant, which makes this pain reliever perfect for your weight loss program. According to an article published in the *African Journal of Biotechnology* in 2006, the Kola nut revs up your metabolism when taken at low concentrations, thus promoting weight loss.

While most pain meds clog your liver, Recovery Agent helps to raise bile production which then helps lessen fatty deposits in the liver, which further relieves joint pain by helping the body metabolize fat better, so it will be easier to lose weight. Milk thistle has been used for over 2,000 years medicinally; it is a related to the daisy and indigenous to the

Mediterranean. Milk thistle includes silymarin (often used interchangeably with milk thistle), an antioxidant which is believed to protect against cell damage. Studies have shown that taking milk thistle can decrease blood sugar levels and improve cholesterol numbers in those with Type 2 diabetes. It has been shown potentially effective in the treatment of seasonal allergies and heartburn (when used in combination with other ingredients).

LEAN SLEEP

I am always working to improve my sleep, as sleep is the secret to losing weight and melting fat, not to mention its critical to the anti-aging process and who doesn't want to slow that down? Sleep is where everything happens. So if you struggle with anything in your life; whether its cravings, losing weight, melting stubborn fat, depression, anxiety, pain (chronic pain) control, injuries, and even medical issues like heart palpitations, diabetes, or high blood sugar—you name it—sleep helps it. Just about every ailment under the sun can be helped by getting better quality sleep and we all know it certainly won't hurt. God very intricately designed your body to heal on its own, and when you're not sleeping, you're not healing. The conditions listed above may not only appear, but they won't go away. Want to feel better fast? Work on your sleep. It's guaranteed to improve whatever ails you.

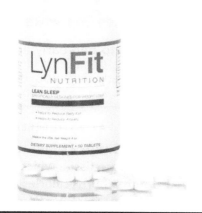

LEAN SLEEP
Suggested Usage: Take one 5 mg tablet 30 to 60 minutes before bedtime to sleep and wake up refreshed. Designed to be dissolved under the tongue for quick absorption, but may be swallowed whole.
LynFit Lean Tip: Take Lean Sleep with you when you travel to help you naturally adjust to different time zones.

Despite its importance, sleep is an often-overlooked factor. Most of us are chronically sleep-deprived due to travel, work schedule, stress, or some other reason. It can be difficult to maintain a healthy weight or to lose weight when lack of sleep is an issue. There is a surefire way to improve your sleep; melatonin, which plays a big role in your body's ability to get to sleep.

What is melatonin? A nonaddicting hormone that the pineal gland in your brain secretes to help regulate other hormones and continue and maintain the circadian rhythm of your body. Under normal conditions our bodies secrete it naturally, but who lives under normal conditions anymore? I always urge my clients to work on lifestyle factors affecting sleep and circadian rhythms (more on this below), but when you can't change your life, you can still change how you sleep.

Your circadian rhythm is the internal clock that helps to determine when you fall asleep and when you wake from sleep. When you don't follow a healthy lifestyle, which includes going to bed early enough for your body to do what it needs to and wake up at the same time every day, you disrupt the natural circadian rhythm of your body and disrupt melatonin production. This creates a need to supplement with melatonin, especially when you are trying to lose weight. Believe it or not, your body is designed to eat dinner around 5pm and be in bed relaxing by sundown (remember, before electricity?). In optimal health, your body is organically created to rise

> **MELT FAT WITH MELATONIN**
>
> MELATONIN IS AN IMPORTANT regulator of brown adipose tissue which is a "good-for-you" fat that burns calories instead of storing them, thereby ramping up the body's metabolism. In the fall of 2013 Spanish scientists published a study in the *Journal of Pineal Research* proving that melatonin promotes such "beige fat."

with the sun—we humans mess with our bodies' organic chemistry by not sticking with this sun-up-to-sun-down plan (realistically it's not feasible in the modern age), and this is the best way to gain weight and cause disease. As you live *The Metabolism Solution*, you will see your sleep improve, and you'll begin feeling rejuvenated with seven hours of sleep—an optimal amount—and you'll wake up feeling refreshed when or even before the sun comes up. I know what you're saying to yourself right now. I, too, was a very late sleeper and struggled with my weight until I began working out in the morning and then amazing things began to happen— and not just to my waistline but in my life.

THE SLEEP DO'S

✓ **DO** stop all stressful activity (this includes loud music and stress-inducing TV) early enough to allow your body to wind down.
✓ **DO** turn down the lights—yep, this includes light from computers, e-readers, and cell phones
✓ **DO** create a sleep-wake schedule so you go to bed and get up the same time every day including weekends. (*It's ok to stay up 1 hour later on weekends BUT anymore creates the issues we are trying to solve)
✓ **DO** take a LynFit Lean Sleep 45 minutes before bedtime or as soon as you remember.

AND DON'TS

• **DON'T** sleep in whatever you do. Need more sleep? Go to bed earlier the following night or take a quick 20-minute nap. A longer nap may mess with your body clock.
• **DON'T** drink alcohol. It is the worst beverage to drink before you go to sleep. Alcohol may make you feel tired, but once it has metabolized in your body, it will wake you up. Stop drinking at least 2 hours before bed to avoid disrupting the natural rhythm necessary for good sleep. Remember alcohol is bad for weight loss.
• **DON'T** eat right before bed. Even a so-called sleep-inducing tryptophan-rich snack is a bad idea. All foods contain many chemicals that affect your body and brain as they are digested. Eating before bed forces your body to do all kinds of work while you're trying to wind down.
• **DON'T** hit the snooze button. There is no benefit to sleeping a few minutes more. While sleeping, you go through different sleep cycles until you reach the restorative kind called REM (rapid eye movement sleep). It takes about 60 minutes to reach that deep, critical sleep cycle and hitting snooze is less than 10 minutes which won't provide what you need anyway. Go to bed earlier instead.
• **DON'T** take other sleep aids. Prescription and the over-the-counter sleep aids as well as all-herbal remedies can slow down your metabolism, impeding your body from releasing those much needed hunger-halting hormones.

Yes, I still have stress and plenty of it, but I feel like I can handle it better and make better conscious decisions that help me move. I never miss my morning workouts anymore, so as a "very-late-I-need-to-sleep-late-I'm-a-night-person-sleeper", I can tell you firsthand it's worth trying this as you won't be sorry and you'll see your life transform before your eyes.

Your body manufactures more melatonin when it is dark and less when it is light. Experiencing bright lights at night (every hour you spend awake past sundown decreases your melatonin) causes you to sleep late, creating a cycle where you can never get enough melatonin. Melatonin is often out of balance in workaholics (like me), night-shift workers, people who travel and have jet lag, and those with poor vision, which affects how their eyes receive sunlight so their bodies

> SUPPLEMENTS are a great alternative to harmful medications that may slow down your metabolism and create more problems than they fix. Switching to alternatives such as Lean Sleep instead of over-the-counter nighttime sleep aids that slow your metabolism is a great way to turn your body into a calorie-burning machine.
>
> Everything we put into out bodies—including medications—can slow your metabolism; all affect your body in one way or another. Smart supplementing boosts you metabolism and turns your body into a thermogenic fat-blasting machine.

can't do their job. And if you're over 40, you can bet your levels are low. Hormonal changes to both women and men as we age affect melatonin as well.

The biggest melatonin drainer? Cell phones and computers. If you're like me and spend way too much time on both late into the night, you are wreaking havoc on your body's melatonin production. And melatonin affects weight in more ways than you can imagine.

> "I lost four inches from my waist and sleep better than I have in years when I switched from over-the-counter sleep-aids to Lean Sleep."   —T.Z.

Most significantly, melatonin alters our sleep patterns and causes sleep deprivation. Harvard Medical School as well as many credible sources including European studies from Spain, Italy, and Sweden, to name but a few, all agree that lack of sleep can affect how your body stores and processes carbohydrates (aka, your metabolism) and can alter levels of certain hormones that affect your appetite such as an increase in the "hunger" hormone ghrelin—the one that makes us

CREATE A SLEEP/WAKE CYCLE TO LOSE WEIGHT BY GOING TO BE AND GETTING UP AT THE SAME TIME EVERYDAY.

hungry. And if that's not bad enough, lack of sleep can also decrease leptin levels, which is the hormone that suppresses hunger. Sleep-deprived people don't crave broccoli, they crave high-fat and high-sugar foods.

Hold on, don't think for one second you can simply take melatonin and continue your late-night-living lifestyle and wake up with washboard abs. It's the lifestyle changes—including diet—and smart usage of melatonin to assist you in learning how to get a good night's sleep again that will bring about lasting changes.

I've seen it time and again in my line of work; the number one reason people can't stick to a regular exercise routine is sleep deprivation. Countless studies show that morning exercisers lose more weight and keep it off compared to those who exercise later in the day. No exercise and eating carbs and fat is a sure way to add to or create a spare tire around your middle. So what can you do to sleep better?

As with diet and exercise, you have to be ready to make the change. It's all a matter of how badly you really

WHY NOT JUST TAKE SLEEPING PILLS?

When you don't get enough sleep, every part of your life can be negatively affected. Insomnia is linked to heart disease and diabetes as well as obesity. And while it might seem convenient to just take a pill, I strongly urge you to consider melatonin instead.

Sleeping pills, be they prescribed or over the counter, do not help with *why* you aren't sleeping. In fact, they are linked to almost a four-time increase in the risk of death and increased cancer risks. According to a study published in February 2012 in BMJ Open, an online medical journal, including more than 10,500 people, "...patients prescribed any hypnotic had substantially elevated hazards of dying compared to those prescribed no hypnotics." Taking as little as 18 sleeping pills a year could increase the average risk.

And unlike melatonin, sleep aids are well-known to potentially leave you still sluggish the next day and can become addictive.

want it. To get over being sick and tired of being sick and tired, I changed my life to revolve around sleep. I have never been happier or felt better. It's completely worth it to me to tell friends (yes, even on weekends) that I need to eat early and get to bed early. My friends understand and support me. Most of them are in the same struggle with weight loss as I am and are happy that I speak up.

SLEEP BETTER— MELT MORE BELLY FAT.

You can, too. Nevertheless, there are always times you cannot change your circumstances—planes are late; kids wake you up; stress hits and keeps you awake; you just have to finish reading the book. I didn't let book deadlines affect my sleep either. I never went to bed later than usual as my life-happiness depends on my being rested, and if I'm not healthy and happy, I cannot do my job effectively. There really are no excuses.

What makes my LynFit Lean Sleep different from any other sleep aid out there is its pure, high-quality melatonin in the amount your body needs to be effective. I don't add inexpensive fillers like B vitamins that could keep you awake or herbs that slow your metabolism down and stop weight loss. The melatonin in it comes from a pharmaceutical lab so you won't find any contaminants that may make

"Lean Sleep helped me stop cravings carbs so I lost weight and feel great."
—*P.R.*

their way into melatonin made from animal sources. Note: Natural isn't always better. In this case, *synthetic* is.

Take one tablet every night, preferably 45 minutes before you bedtime so your brain has time to catch up with your melatonin levels. If you forget to take it at the time interval, it's okay to take it as soon as you remember. Lean Sleep can also be taken in the middle of the night, unlike other sleep agents, and won't leave you groggy the next day.

RASPBERRY KETONE CLEANSE

What could possibly be better for fat loss than raspberry ketones? Raspberry Ketones mixed with African mango. African mango and raspberry ketones help turbo charge your weight loss by cleansing and detoxing your system so it is primed for fat burning. Technically, it's not an African mango but the *Irvingia gabonensis* tree which produces this mango-looking fruit. While the fleshy fruit is eaten all over Africa, it's the seed that's of interest here. It was initially studied for its cholesterol-lowering properties, but found that it could help in weight loss too. The soluble fiber found in the seed has been shown to slow digestion and glucose absorption. According to studies, individuals had significant improvements in their body weight, body fat, and waist size.

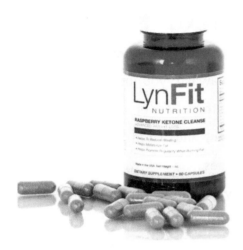

RASPBERRY KETONE CLEANSE
Suggested Usage: This product is formulated to be taken on an occasional basis for no more than 7 days in a row to help cleanse the colon and promote regularity. Take one capsule at 9 a.m. and one capsule at 2 p.m. with at least 8 oz. of water (or as directed by your healthcare practitioner) to burn fat all day.
 LynFit Lean Tip: Take all three capsules at night to reboot or before a bad meal.

This dynamic duo promotes weight loss by speeding up the body's metabolism. Toxins block the body's ability to absorb the proper nutrients and energy needed to burn fat and increase metabolism. When this happens, your metabolism slows down to a screeching halt and fat burning stops. Clogged systems simply do not work properly. When African mango extract is ingested, it eliminates nutrient-blocking toxins which allow the body to acquire the energy it needs to burn fat. Also, in terms of weight loss, the African mango contains loads of vitamin B, which helps to increase metabolism and prompts the body to use carbohydrates, proteins, and fats for fuel instead of storing them. This is how a clean-running system should work. You'll have more energy—you may even want to exercise—which leads to increased fat burning. African mango and raspberry ketones both affect our adiponectin, the amino acid that regulates how your body absorbs glucose and increases blood flow for better circulation. Better circulation always means better fat loss, especially from those stubborn hard to reach places like the thighs, buttocks, and abs.

The Raspberry Ketone Cleanse promotes regularity for optimal health and faster weight loss, with health benefits including; overall colon health, internal cleansing, reduced bloating, and prevention of occasional constipation due to dietary changes.

> **THE 10-STEP 48-HOUR METABOLIC-BOOSTING RASPBERRY KETONE CLEANSE**
>
> 1) Aim to sleep 7 to 8 hours per night
> 2) Drink 8 to 10 glasses of water daily
> 3) EAT 10 servings of veggies daily and cabbage is king for cleansing
> 4) Take 1 Raspberry Ketone Cleanse capsule 3 times a day for 2 days
> 5) Perform metabolic boosting exercise 3 days per week to turbocharge your metabolism and walk as much as possible
> 6) Allow yourself to be hungry. It's a sign that your body is burning fat
> 7) Drop all other supplements except the ones suggested.
> 8) Eat foods from approved list only.
> 9) Drink your coffee or tea black only
> 10) Use only LynFit shakes and meal replacement lean bars as they are the only ones designed to boost your metabolism

THE DAILY POWER SHOT

If I could bottle motivation it would be the Daily Power Shot. It is the best way to take your multiple vitamins and minerals every day. In fact, some of the nutrients included in the Daily Power Shot are so special that they used to be available only by injection—before a liquid form was available. Thankfully there's no need for that anymore.

Weight control is an essential aspect of good health and most of us even know what to do—so why don't we do it? I'm convinced it's because we do not feel good; we lack the energy to even remember what it was we were supposed to do, let alone do it. One of the

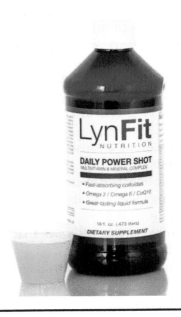

things we lack energy for? Exercise. Who feels like exercising regularly all the time? I feel too exhausted to exercise at times thanks to all I do for the kids, my husband, the dogs, work, and all the mundane things that make up our lives. I've looked enviously at those women who seem to be able to do it all. Have you? What makes them tick? Energy. Energy to do it all, and that changes everything. You need a jumpstart of good sound healthy energy.

DAILY POWER SHOT
Suggested Usage: 1 ounce once or twice daily as desired. Recommended for anyone who is on a weight loss or fitness program, under stress, or interested in adding key nutrients related to improving heart health.
LynFit Lean Tip: Take 30 minutes before you work out or at 7 a.m.

Daily Power Shot is loaded with 90 essential nutrients and 60 different trace minerals so your body gets everything it needs to be energized and healthy. Because it's a liquid in colloidal form, Daily Power Shot works immediately—you won't have to wait for the energy because the nutrients within the Daily Power Shot are absorbed more easily and rapidly and provide instant energy, letting you do the things you need to do. You'll crave less because your body will be nourished the right way, with every nutrient it needs to stay healthy.

"I was taking too many pills every day for chronic fatigue. Once I started taking Power Shot as my multivitamin, I could take less medicine." —J.D.

Taking the Power Shot daily provides your body with the right amounts of vitamins and minerals as well as important enzymes, and it gives your body the nutritional support it needs for maximum efficiency and optimal metabolic support making weight loss easier. The chemical reactions involved in metabolism require the raw materials, which the Daily Power Shot provides.

Starting your day with the Power Shot affects your metabolism, and your life, more than you know. The Daily Power Shot with its vitamins and minerals act as as a catalyst to speed reactions that result in weight loss. For instance, the B vitamins found in Power Shot are essential for the metabolism of proteins and carbohydrates. Vitamin B12 aids in red blood cell formation, which deliver oxygen to the body. If you exercise to lose weight, an increase in red blood cells can increase your endurance by increasing your body's efficiency in producing energy and leaving you feeling good.

"I was relying on store-bought energy drinks to pick me up and found myself feeling worse. Now my kids can't keep up with me." —C.K.

It amazes me that our bodies produce no minerals. None. Even though the body can produce some of the vitamins required, it cannot do the same for minerals. Yet minerals are necessary for 95 percent of the body's daily functions, especially when it comes to weight loss and working out. When you work out your body requires more nutrients. And if you lack even minute amounts of certain minerals, you may suffer from muscle pain, weakness, a slow thyroid, slow wound healing, or hair loss. To add to it, when you lack certain minerals even vitamins have a reduced effectiveness and the entire weight loss process, your metabolism, can be slowed to a crawl. You find yourself out of energy and just feeling yucky.

DID YOU KNOW YOUR BODY DOESN'T MAKE MINERALS? SUPPLEMENT DAILY WITH LIQUID POWER SHOT TO GET YOURS.

Supplementing daily with the Daily Power shot is the best way to ensure that vitamins and minerals are present at the same time for health and wellness and when trying to lose weight. Absorption is key and that's what makes a liquid form better than a tablet. It takes longer for your body to absorb vitamins and minerals in tablet form than in liquid. And therefore it takes longer for you to feel the positive effect. With my Power Shot you feel better right away—and who doesn't want that?

Why is Power Shot better than all of the rest? It is all natural and suspended in a liquid base of papaya that helps vitamins and minerals be absorbed faster—and it's delicious. Because of the colloidal minerals' microscopic size and because of their suspension in liquid form, they are absorbed through the walls of the intestine and colon at a much greater rate than mineral in tablet form. Over 90 essential nutrients, including over 60 different trace minerals, along with 100 percent RDA of vitamins as well as the superstar ingredients are included. The best thing isn't just what's in Daily Power Shot, but rather what's not. You won't find any harmful junk found in over-the-counter stimulants that cause jitters. There's also no red food dye or sugar—like you'll find in some popular store brands—that could hurt your metabolism.

> VITAMIN D IS NECESSARY FOR BONES AND MORE. A STUDY IN SHOWS THAT LOW LEVELS OF IT MEAN THE HORMONE LEPTIN, WHICH TELLS THE BRAIN YOU ARE FULL, DOESN'T WORK AS IT SHOULD.

Power Shot is loaded with superstar ingredients. If you've read about it or seen it on television, it's in there. I put these high-quality superstars in exactly the amount needed in a super-easy way to take so you need less and save money.

It's fitting that vitamins dominate Power Shot because several of them play a key role in metabolism. Take vitamin A. Like vitamin B12, it supports red blood cell formation in the body. Vitamin A also assists in the removal of free radicals produced from oxygen metabolism. Vitamin B2 helps the body use oxygen more efficiently. Biotin and pantothenic acid support healthy carbohydrate metabolism. The combined action of these B's aid weight loss by allowing your body to properly metabolize and process the foods you eat.

Biotin is essential for your metabolic process. This vitamin processes nearly every type of food that you ingest, including carbohydrates, protein, and fat. When biotin is at the proper level in your body, the food that you take in will be processed quickly. Your doctor may even prescribe a biotin supplement if you suffer from metabolic issues, since it can help get your metabolism up to normal functioning levels quickly. If you are trying to lose weight, a biotin supplement may help, since it is sometimes thought to speed up weight loss, due to its clear effects on metabolic levels.

Biotin also plays a major role in your blood glucose production. Since it is heavily involved in the breakdown of carbohydrates within your body, it is largely responsible for keeping your blood sugar at healthy levels.

Folic acid is part of the B vitamin family and is known as vitamin B-9. It is absolutely crucial for pregnant women as it reduces a baby's risk for birth defects in the brain (anencephaly) and spine (spina bifida) by 50 to 70 percent. It can be found in green, leafy foods; beans, peas, and lentils; and lemons, bananas, and melons. It is often added to fortified baked goods, as required by federal law. Your body needs folic acid to make and maintain cells to create the very DNA that makes you, you.

PLACE POWER SHOT FRONT AND CENTER IN YOUR REFRIGERATOR SO YOU NEVER FORGET.

Folic acid helps in the prevention of Type 2 diabetes by helping with the breakdown of triglycerides (bad fat) in the blood. It also helps metabolize proteins for energy. Combined with vitamins B-12 and C, it helps you keep stable blood sugar levels, which helps with fat burning.

Vitamin D is necessary for bone health, but it also boosts your immune system and plays a role as an anti-inflammatory agent. Vitamin D might even help lessen symptoms of mild depression. People who are overweight often have lower levels of vitamin D. A study in the United Kingdom at the Aberdeen University Department of Medicine and Therapeutics in 2008 established that low levels of vitamin D meant that the hormone leptin, which tells the brain you are full, didn't work as it should. So if you're body is telling you it's still hungry you may overeat. This particular study found that obese people have up to 10 percent less

Vitamin D than those of average weight and this excess fat absorbed the Vitamin D, stopping it from doing its job in the body. Another British study (published in the *British Journal of Nutrition* in 2008) ascertained that those with more Vitamin D when on a diet lost more weight and fat.

The best natural source of vitamin D is sunlight. 10 to 15 minutes a week of sun exposure without sunscreen may give you enough vitamin D, but most of us can't (or won't risk skin cancer) manage that—and sometimes mother nature doesn't cooperate. While fortified foods (milk) often contain vitamin D, and some foods have amounts of it as well (such as fish and eggs), it's best to get it in a supplement as your body absorbs it better.

Many of the vitamins supporting metabolism and weight loss are water-soluble. This means that they are not stored in great quantities in your body. Therefore, to get the greatest benefit of vitamins for weight loss, you should stay on a regular schedule of taking these supplements.

Minerals play a key role in Power Shot, too. Daily Power Shot provides 100 percent of the RDA recommended dose of magnesium and chromium. Many chemical reactions involved in metabolism depend on magnesium. It is also required for the formation of adenosine triphosphate—ATP—a synthesizing protein. ATP is the energy currency of the human body. It is required by every cell to function. Chromium is specifically involved with sugar metabolism. It helps maintain normal blood sugar levels by enhancing the effects of insulin.

You'll also find ginkgo biloba in the Power Shot. Ginkgo biloba is one of the top-selling herbs in the United States. It has been used in traditional medicines for thousands of years. Ginkgo is full of antioxidant flavonoids, similar to those found in green tea, which have been linked to boosting weight loss.

Grape seed extract is another powerful antioxidant I put in the Power Shot. You may be familiar with grape seed extract because it is used in many topical skincare products to help reduce signs of aging, such as wrinkles. Grape seed extract, which can be made from the byproducts of wine production, helps from the inside as well. It is an anti-inflammatory and benefits circulation by helping with the breakdown of fats in the blood.

Cat's claw, also known as Una de Gato is included for its anti-inflammatory, anti-viral, and anti-bacterial benefits. This South American herbal plant has been used for centuries in Peru for all kinds of ailments. It is a powerful immune booster.

The Daily Power Shot includes CoQ10 (Coenzyme Q-10), another popular supplement of late. It is naturally occurring in the body, but decreases as we age; therefore, it is beneficial to supplement. CoQ10 produces energy and boosts metabolism while serving as a powerful antioxidant that's good for fighting signs of aging on the skin.

Quercitin is a high-powered flavonoid, an anti-inflammatory and antioxidant that helps boost metabolism—that's why it's in the Power Shot. Quercitin has been used to treat high blood pressure and shows promise in anti-cancer treatments. It is found in apples and onions and in many fruits and vegetables. Eating more quercitin-laced food has shown decreased risks of various cancers. New studies show promise for quercitin to treat stress-related conditions as well.

Quercitin is proving to be highly beneficial for weight loss. It boosts adiponectin levels in the body which helps you metabolize glucose efficiently. And what makes quercitin really special is that a study showed it blocks development of new fat cells in the body by up to 70 percent.

Finally, I want to discuss selenium. This essential mineral is found in the soil and in water and plays a vital role in your body's metabolic process. Nuts and fish are foods high in selenium. Your body needs a minute amount of this mineral to regulate the thyroid, which in turn regulates your body's hormones affecting how fat, protein, and carbs are used.

Studies on selenium and cancer have shown promise. Several studies associate low levels of selenium with an increased risk of cancer death. A Malaysian study published in the *Singapore Medical Journal* in 2009 showed a link between low selenium levels and breast cancer in particular.

If you have suffered with hyperthyroidism as I have, selenium is a must. Not only does it give your immune system a boost, it helps your metabolism. Supplementing is crucial as most of us do not get enough from our food. Combine that with poor food choices and dieting, which creates a demand for more, and supplements become critical.

LISA'S SUPPLEMENT SCHEDULE

- **Within one hour of waking up, usually between 5 and 6 a.m., I have a Complete Protein shake.**

- **30 minutes before I work out I take the Daily Power Shot and Cutting Edge.**

- **Immediately after my workout I take Pure Omega-3 and another Cutting Edge.**

- **With lunch I take a Carb Edge.**

- **At 3 p.m. I take another Carb Edge and Pure Omega-3.**

- **3 hours before bed (usually around 7); I take a Raspberry Ketone Cleanse when I feel the need.**

- **30 minutes before going to bed I take one Lean Sleep.**

I'll take an additional Power Shot if and when needed or if I feel like I'm feeling sick I'll take Recovery Agent. For special occasions and bathing suit season, I add Accelerator.

Four

THERMOGENIC EATING FOR RADICAL WEIGHT LOSS

Every day I get emails from desperate people who have tried every diet on the planet and yet they just can't seem to lose weight. Getting your body to switch over from fat-storing mode to fat-burning mode is easier than you think. Food is the problem *and the answer*. And the solution is right in your refrigerator—or what's *not* in your refrigerator. So how do we get our bodies to switch from weight gain to weight loss while keeping our calories high enough? By eating the right metabolism-boosting, thermogenic foods.

"Thermogenic" is an up and coming word in nutrition these days. It describes foods that take almost as many calories (or more) to digest as they put into the body. These foods increase the metabolism after you eat them.

Every single bite you put in your mouths counts and affects whether you gain or lose. *Every* bite. Even a small micro dot of a bite has an effect on blood sugar, which is more sensitive than you can imagine. Before you put anything in your mouth, ask yourself; will this food enhance my metabolism or slow it down? Eating only a "little" of a metabolism-slowing food will stop weight loss in its tracks.

The Metabolism Solution is all about super-charging your metabolism. Every food you eat or don't, every supplement you take, your metabolic workout—all provide a super-charge to your metabolism and get it burning like crazy so you can begin losing weight immediately. The more good choices you make daily, the faster you'll lose weight. Guaranteed!

Every time you skip drinking a Complete Protein Shake or eating a Lean Bar (other shakes and lean bars will not work the same), eat chicken when you're supposed to have fish, skimp on the veggies, or don't drink enough water, you slow down your metabolism. If you eat protein that's high in fat like red meat, pork (it's *not* the other white meat), or processed meats such as sausage or bacon (yes, even turkey bacon), and the so-called healthy grains sold in gourmet markets, you are slowing down your metabolism. Just because a food may be good for you, doesn't mean it's good for weight loss—especially if you have more than 10 pounds to lose. What to avoid then? Breads, rice, all pasta, chips, crackers, starchy vegetables like potatoes, butternut squash, oatmeal, and basically any food you don't see listed on my metabolic-boosting food lists that follow. Watch out for the diet-*deceptor* foods: avocados; nuts and oils (we eat too many); all nut butters; cheese, soy, almond, and coconut milks as well as all nondairy creamers (even the nonfat ones). These are usually the foods that keep you from losing weight in the first place. But don't worry—this book is full of delicious replacements for everything you crave. And in time your cravings will stop, and you'll be leaner and feel better in no time at all—it's a guarantee.

The Metabolism Solution fixes these problems by re-booting your metabolism in a healthy way with wholesome, clean, fat-burning foods that supercharge your metabolism every time you eat them. And did I mention that these foods deliver powerful nutrients so you'll feel better fast? A clean food is one that is close to its natural state, not overly processed, not filled with loads of preservatives or added sugar, and no high levels of bad fats (some saturated fats and all trans fats). What is a "clean" calorie? One that is free of saturated fats and derived from a natural source.

EVERYTHING YOU HAVE BEEN TAUGHT ABOUT EATING FOR WEIGHT LOSS IS ALL WRONG

When it comes to good nutrition, the one thing all experts agree on is that food is The Holy Grail for good health. The best way to get what you need is through your diet. But when it comes to boosting your metabolism, everything you have been taught is all wrong. Not all clean foods are Thermogenic. I'll give you an example: Potatoes can be considered a clean food, yet they can slow weight loss due to the rise in your blood sugar. Other clean vegetables, like broccoli, for instance, increase your metabolism after you eat them.

Take carbohydrates, for another example. I hear you now, "But doesn't my body need carbs?" Yes, but not the kind of carbs you're thinking. Carbs are by and large responsible for our nation's obesity issues. The nutrients we need from carbohydrate sources can all be found in vegetables. (Carbs, however, do come in handy when you're trying to keep weight on; so if you lose weight too fast, I always suggest adding a small carb serving back into your diet.) In fact, our bodies are now extremely resistant to weight loss and fat loss—specifically from the belly area—because we over eat on this food group. And just because some carbs come from the earth doesn't mean they're good for metabolic boosting.

Same goes for foods labeled low-fat or nonfat. While they may be low-fat, they don't always give you that metabolic boost because they may spike blood sugar. In fact, most low-fat and nonfat foods are loaded with sugar. Not good for weight loss.

There are foods that you must avoid if you are trying to lose weight. To make it simple, I'm going to give you a list of what you *can* eat. If you don't see it on the lists, don't eat it. I urge you to memorize the lists so you never succumb to food temptation. And remember, drinking a protein shake has you losing weight right away, and one of its added benefits is that it helps you keep losing even while you learn (sometimes through trial and error) what you can and cannot eat when losing weight. Think of a shake as a little extra weight loss insurance.

The secret solution to boosting the metabolism is lowering blood sugar levels. That's why what you eat is 80 percent; nope, scratch that, more like *90 percent* of your weight loss success—especially if you're female and over 40 or have a damaged metabolism. What you *don't* eat makes all the difference. It's really not as simple as calories in and calorie's out—especially if you have a stubborn metabolism. If it were this simple, we would all simply eat what we want and count calories until we reach our daily limit. If you're reading this book, you've probably already tried that method with little success.

The Metabolism Solution is the healthiest diet of them all—it's the Ferrari of all plans; gluten-free, alkalinizing, low-carb, low-sugar, and low-fat. You cannot find a healthier and easier way to live. On my plan I will not tell you that you can never ever eat a certain food again. You won't starve, you won't feel weak. You will eat.

LEAN, CLEAN PROTEIN

Protein is the foundation of *The Metabolism Solution*. It stabilizes blood sugar levels, which helps to curb cravings, and feeds your muscles, speeding up your metabolism. But I'm not talking any old protein—sirloin steak does not make the cut. The proteins eaten on *The Metabolism Solution* are chosen for their ability to elevate your metabolism. They have the right nutrients to do just that.

> THE LIGHTER AND WHITER THE FISH THE BETTER FOR YOUR METABOLISM

You may have seen me on *Dr. Oz* talking about specific types of fish that enhance metabolism. My line that gets quoted all the time was; "The lighter and

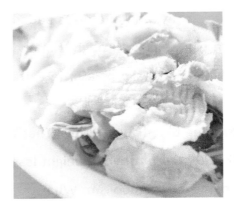

whiter the fish the better for your metabolism." Dr. Oz was in full agreement. White fish is lower in calories and extremely low in bad fat when compared to other fattier fish like salmon and swordfish. Salmon and swordfish are not *bad* for you, a whiter fish is *better*. The whiter the fish the faster you'll lose weight. Why? It's lower in calories and fat, making it very Thermogenic. Stick to fattier fish (and this includes poultry, too) to one to two times a week, and make sure to weigh out your portion since even a slight increase of one ounce can slow down your weight loss. If you find you're not losing at the pace you want, cut down even more on the fattier fish and switch to lighter, whiter fish.

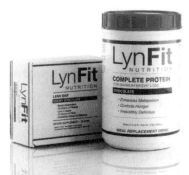

The best choice you can make when it comes to protein is the LynFit Complete Protein Shake. Right alongside it is my Lean Bar. Note: You cannot buy a better protein bar for weight loss. My bars are the only ones out there made with the same high-grade protein that goes into my protein powder. This high-grade whey can raise the metabolism by 25% contains every amino acid (in predigested form—to make it easier for the body to use and to avoid gastric distress) that your body needs. However, it is important to vary your diet.

THREE TO FOUR PROTEINS A DAY TAKE THE POUNDS AWAY

Complete Protein Shake (2 per day max.)	Tuna Fresh or Canned 3 oz.
LynFit Lean Bar (2 per day max.)	Mahi-Mahi 4 oz.
Egg Whites (3 to 4)	Clams 4 oz.
Scrod/Cod 4 oz.	Mussels 4 oz.
Flounder 4 oz.	Oysters 5 oz.
Haddock 4 oz.	Crab 4 oz.
Halibut 4 oz.	Lobster 1 ½ lb (whole)
Scallops 4 oz.	Calamari 4-5 oz.
Orange Roughly 4 oz.	Salmon 4 oz.
Grouper 4 oz.	Swordfish 4 oz.
Tilapia 4 oz.	Sashimi 4 oz.
Shrimp 4 oz. (shelled)	Sardines 3 oz.
Sea Bass 4 oz.	Herring 4 oz.
Snapper 4 oz. (all)	Trout/Rainbow Trout 4 oz.
Mussels 4 oz	Sashimi 4 oz.
Chicken Breast 3 oz. (no skin)*	Turkey Breast 3 oz. (no skin)*
Nonfat Cottage Cheese 1/2 cup	

Start your day with a shake for breakfast and try to eat fish once per day along with other sources of protein such as egg whites. By varying your protein sources, you gain varied nutrient benefits while stimulating your metabolism.

Learn the list of proteins on page 89, which are in order of their preference for weight loss. Remember, a serving is 3 to 4 ounces. Teens and men (sorry ladies) can increase portions to 4 to 5 ounces each. Enjoy these baked, broiled, grilled, or steamed (without butter or skin). Aim for three to four servings per day (unless noted). And if you find you're one of the lucky ones who lose weight fast, add an ounce to your portion.

THE RIGHT CARBOHYDRATES: SUPER VEGGIES FOR SUPER FAST FAT LOSS

If you're like me and you like to eat a lot of food but need to keep your calories low in order to lose weight, vegetables are the key to your success. Don't like to eat your veggies? Keep

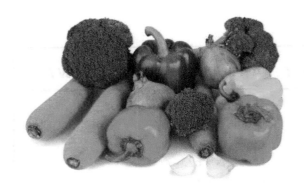

trying different kinds and be sure to check out the recipes in this book. My vegetable recipes won't make you feel like you're denying yourself. The best thing about veggies, (especially fibrous carbohydrates like those listed on page 93)? They are nutrient-rich and will leave you full and satisfied because of their high fiber content, decreasing your appetite and helping to eliminate cravings for high-sugar foods. These good-for-you carbs slow down the digestive process which helps rev up your metabolism. Fiber, while not absorbed by your body, grabs fatty acids and other unwanted objects as it passes through helping them pass through your system. Think of fiber as a sponge that absorbs unwanted and unhealthy material while scouring your insides clean. Clean intestines let your body absorb more nutrients and vitamins, be they from diet or supplement. Constipation, a clogged system, feels horrible, so you must eat enough vegetables to ensure adequate fiber. Another plus for these fibrous carb wonders; they speed your liver's cleansing process, which is important for optimal health, most especially when losing body fat.

Vegetables are the main source of carbohydrates on *The Metabolism Solution*. Because most of us cannot spend 20 hours a week exercising to combat insulin resistance and working off the effects of a starchy diet, we need to eat lower amounts of starchy carbohydrates. That's why focusing on veggies is the solution to your weight loss. Vegetables are lower in calories and you can eat larger portions while still losing weight. By eating more veggies, you minimize your body's demand for insulin and lower your cells' resistance to its effects.

> WE ALL KNOW that carbs such as bread, pasta, crackers, and of course all of the refined carbohydrates such as cookies, cakes, and candies are not good for weight loss, BUT even the so-called "healthy grains" such as rice, oatmeal, potatoes, and any other carbohydrate (even if its gourmet and found in a health food store) is not going to help you boost your metabolism. Keep it simple. Remember: If it's not found on the vegetable list, it's a starchy carbohydrate and will cause your insulin to spike and stop weight loss instantly. Even the tiniest of servings.

These fibrous carbohydrates are not the carbs you need to worry about. They are what I like to call "free food" as most of us don't overeat on vegetables—we typically don't eat enough.

Only the vegetables on my list (page 93) are the metabolism miracles. Eating enough of these vegetables is *the* solution to boosting your metabolism (along with lean proteins of course), and if you don't eat enough of them, you slow your metabolism down. Without butter or oil, your body actually uses more calories just to digest them than they contain so you practically end up with a caloric deficit. That's exactly

> WARNING: THIS DIET CAUSES FAST WEIGHT LOSS AND CREATES HEALTH QUICKLY.

what you want when you're trying to lose weight. All foods have some calories or energy, and all foods also require some energy by the body to burn them. It's at this point that the concept of the "negative calorie" comes in. If a food requires more of the body's energy to

DRESS YOUR SALAD LEAN

When I first began trying to lose weight, I switched from hamburgers to salads and couldn't figure out why I wasn't losing weight. I made a common mistake, one you've probably made before, too: My salads were often as calorie-laden as a hamburger with all the foods I put in them. Just because it's called a "Salad" doesn't mean it's good for you. Beans, cheese, and egg yolks may be delicious, but they are higher in fat and calories than a burger and fries. Salads need to be delicious and simple, clean, to satisfy while boosting your metabolism. My suggestion: Stick with the lists on these pages.

I avoid bottled dressings by putting vinegar in a spray bottle and misting my salads to coat them evenly and efficiently—no oils. I'm also a big fan of laying HOT fish or chicken on top and letting the juices seep down over my food—then I don't even need dressing.

What should you do when you're out at a restaurant? Either ask the waiter for a vinegar, bring your own, or you can always mix mustard with balsamic vinegar (add 1 Splenda or Truvia if needed) for a delicious dressing or sauce. If you just cannot eat salad or veggies without dressing? That's okay, you'll get there sooner than you think. In the meantime, find your favorite dressing in a fat-free formulation, or the lowest fat and calories you can find. Try cutting it with some vinegar. But let me be honest: It's better to eat salads with a little dressing than to never eat salads at all. If this is what you need to do to get your veggies in—Do whatever it takes until you can bare them in a dryer state.

There's nothing better than fresh greens with fresh lemon juice and salt and pepper on top.

Salad need crunch? Add lightly cooked veggies or cut up carrots to add crunch without loading up on calories, and egg whites are a good addition just leave off the yolk.

Try replacing the oils in your dressings with fat-free chicken broth. It has almost the same slinky texture without the calories.

adequately burn than the food actually produces, then that food helps create a real Thermogenic effect. As the theory goes, you can eat negative calorie foods to your heart's content and never gain weight. Not only that—you'll lose weight. Vegetables are "careful carbs" that won't affect weight loss unless you don't eat *enough* of them. If you're not losing weight fast enough, you're probably not eating enough vegetables ("careful carbs"). Vegetables are the only food group we do not eat enough of. Thermogenic fibrous carbs cause your metabolism to speed up. Combine this with eating clean following *The Metabolism Solution* and your body will incinerate calories at a fat-burning rate. If you've been following the plan exactly, I guarantee it.

You must eat at least five servings (1/2 cup, unless otherwise noted) a day of these metabolic miracles. Ten is even better. Fibrous carbohydrates like these listed also speed your liver's cleansing process, which is very important for optimal health, especially when losing body fat. Enjoy them steamed, raw, fresh, frozen, or canned—if you must. Just be sure to rinse them thoroughly. I always aim for organic. And remember; *do not* add any fats. No butter, no oil. Try sprinkling your vegetables with lemon juice and a pinch of salt and/or pepper. Or try a dash of Balsamic or apple cider vinegar.

Carbohydrates can be quite nutritious, but they do affect blood sugar levels more than any other food group because we over-eat them. Have belly fat? It's a sign you're eating too many carbs. The solution? Cut back. Especially on bread and crackers until you reach your goal weight. And be sure to check labels; carbs sneak in everywhere. Be on guard for any

---

TEN VEGGIES A DAY MELT THE FAT AWAY

Alfalfa Sprouts	Collard Greens	Radishes
Asparagus	Cucumbers	Spinach
Broccoflower	Eggplant	Tomato Juice (4 oz.)
Broccoli	Escarole	Tomatoes*
Brussels Sprouts	Green Beans	Yellow Beans
Cabbage (all types)	Kale	Yellow Squash
Carrots	Lettuces (all;	Wax Beans
Cauliflower	serving is 3 cups)	Zucchini
Celery	Onion	

Tomatoes are technically a fruit, so IF you are extremely insulin-sensitive or your body is acidic, eat less until desired weight loss is achieved.

---

other brand of protein shake or protein bar. Many of them contain low-quality carbs—especially sugar—because they are inexpensive to use.

Not all carbs are created equal. Vegetable sources are the best and cleanest form of carbohydrates when it comes to boosting your stubborn metabolism. If you are one of the lucky ones who have low body fat and can eat some carbs and keep your weight in check, you can skip this and continue eating carbs the way you always have. But if you want to eat as healthily as possible, choose carbs that come from the earth for optimal health and nutrients. Yes, carbs can be part of healthy diet, but if you have ever been overweight and specifically need to lose excess belly and/or thigh fat, this is your body's way of letting you know you need to cut back on carbs—and this may or may not include fruits and any carbs found in yogurts or pre-packaged food. It's best and quickest to eliminate carbs while your belly gets lean.

THE NOT-SO THERMOGENIC CARBS

While these foods may be considered healthy, they also spike blood sugar levels which slows the weight loss process. The bottom line? The less carbs you eat the faster you will lose weight. But if you need or choose select from below.

All Bran (1/2 cup)	**Corn (1/2 cup)**	**Rice Bran (1/2 cup)**
Barley (1/2 cup)	**Fiber One cereal (1/2 cup)**	**Sweet Potato (1/2 cup)**
Beans—Black, Fava, Garbanzo, Kidney, Lentils, Lima, Northern, Pinto, Red, Soy, White (2 TBSP)	**Oatmeal (slow cooking, 1/2 cup)**	**Wasa Light (1 piece)**
Beets (1/2 cup)	**Parsnips (1/2 cup)**	**Whole Grain Breads (1 oz.)**
Brown or Wild Rice (1/2 cup)	**Pasta (1/2 cup)** **Peas (1/2 cup)** **Popcorn (air popped, 3 cups)**	**Winter Squash (all varieties, 1/2 cup)**

Your brain does run on carbs and it does need glucose for fuel to function properly, and it can and will get them from the foods you eat on *The Metabolism Solution*. If you're following this plan, eating an apple every day, and loading up on veggies, you'll be lean in no time and your body will get the carbohydrates it needs to function and fuel your body and brain.

When you over-eat carbohydrates; say like when you eat out and have more than half a cup of pasta, a piece of bread, and dessert, your body pumps out insulin, a hormone to keep your blood sugar within a certain range (otherwise your brain would go haywire). Insulin is also a powerful fat-storage hormone, so your body stores the excess sugar *as fat* (especially under stressful conditions when your cortisol levels are high). Go ahead, take a look at your middle. Are you storing excess fat in this area? It doesn't matter how healthy you're eating when you overload on carbs—even the gourmet "health" carb of the month like quinoa. Once you replace your current diet with lean proteins and vegetables, your stomach will disappear quickly and you'll lose weight easily.

What separates the good carbs from the bad? When it comes to boosting your metabolism all carbohydrates, only those that come from a vegetable (high-fiber) source fit the bill. We only need one-third of the calories we eat every day and reducing the bad carbs is the fastest way to do that. I'm sorry to be the bearer of this news (don't shoot the messenger), but as America gets fatter each minute and unhealthier due to the rise in

---

WHAT'S IT GOING TO BE: WINE OR YOUR WAISTLINE?

Alcohol (a carb) and fat loss don't mix. Refrain from drinking *any* alcoholic beverages when boosting your metabolism. Your waistline will be glad you did and you'll feel better. I am always asked how to work alcohol into my diet. The answer is simple. Sorry, you can't. Alcohol is second only to dietary fat when it comes to useless calories—not to mention it lowers your resolve so you end up eating more calories due to the blood sugar dips. Doesn't matter if it's clear or organic. Show me a fat stomach and I'll show you a drinker. I recommend not having *any* until you reach goal weight, and once you arrive, if you insist, have one glass of wine weekly. When alcohol passes the liver it produces a byproduct called acetate which inhibits fat-burning capabilities –the whole purpose of my plan is to rev up your metabolism.

Your body cannot store calories from alcohol for later, the way it does with calories from food. When you drink, your metabolism slows down or stops what it is doing (like burning off the calories form your last meal or what you're eating while your drinking) to get rid of the booze. Drinking presses the pause button on your metabolism, pushes away other calories, and says "break me down first". The result? What you most recently ate got stored as fat.

---

blood-sugar levels, I have to tell you the truth: You need to cut down on non-vegetable carbs. You especially need to cut down on carbohydrates as you age and your lack of activity

SUGAR SUBSTITUTES: THE FACTS WITHOUT ALL THE HYPE

Did you know that the average American consumes 3 pounds of sugar a week? Blame sugar for obesity, hypertension, fatigue, high blood pressure, headaches, and the metabolic meltdown we are facing in this country. Sugar is as addictive as cocaine.

If you're trying to lose weight, shed belly fat, or just eat healthier, you know that reducing the amount of sugar you eat is one of the most important steps in the process. So when you want something sweet, where do you turn? Artificial sweeteners or other sugar substitutes.

There are pros and cons when it comes to using sugar substitutes, artificial and natural-based. I'm not a proponent of using them, but I'm also not against using artificial sweeteners in moderation. I find it helpful to have a diet soda instead of a bag of "gourmet health chips"—I feel a lot less guilt.

Some top brands you can find today include:

- AGAVE NECTAR comes from the agave plant and is sweeter than honey. Use carefully as it is very high in fructose, which can super-spike blood sugar.
- EQUAL was the first aspartame sweetener sold to the public, hitting the market in 1981. Aspartame safety has been debated over the years, but research studies deem it fine for use.
- NUTRASWEET is another aspartame sweetener.
- SPLENDA is a sucralose-based sweetener that hit the U.S. market in 1999. It is the leading brand in the United States with 60 percent of the sugar-substitute market. Sucralose does not affect blood sugar and it is what I use in my Complete Protein.
- SWEET'N LOW is a saccharin-based sugar substitute. Saccharin has fallen out of favor after some research from the 1970s linked it to cancer in rats. According to the National Cancer Institute, however, subsequent studies have not proven a connection.
- TRUVIA is stevia-based sweetener. Stevia is a South American plant and was approved as a general-use sugar substitute in 2008. In studies, it did not affect blood sugar of those with Type 2 Diabetes or healthy people. Truvia is now the #2 sugar substitute in the United States after Splenda.

You'll find that these 0-calorie sweeteners pop up everywhere and in so many products. (Technically, these sweeteners are not 0 calories. The FDA allows companies to market their products as having "0 calories" if they are 5 calories or less.) But are they good for weight loss? Are they good for you? Well, they don't cause tooth decay and cavities. And many of these synthetic sugars, which have a sweeter taste than actual sugar, have been in use for quite some time without ill effect—diabetics rely on them. There are many research studies confirming their general safety in limited quantities. Using sugar substitutes is an individual choice. Do what's right for you.

decreases. Your body doesn't process carbs the same at 45 as it did at 25. So skip the carbs. If you eat them, take your Carb Edge right before to block 65 percent of unwanted carbohydrates from being broken down into sugar and stored as fat. And if you really must eat your carbs, be sure to always eat it with a lean protein to slow down the carbs from being broken down into sugars.

> **WE ONLY NEED ONE-THIRD OF THE CALORIES WE EAT EVERY DAY. REDUCING CARBS IS THE FASTEST WAY TO DO THAT.**

A LITTLE FAT IS ALL YOU NEED

Yes, you do need fat, but not as much as you may think. When it comes to losing weight, we need less because we already have enough stored. A woman needs about 15 grams of fat a day, a man and teenagers both get 20 grams. This is where most people get stymied in their weight loss because they are unaware of where fats lurk in food. And just because a fat is good for you, doesn't mean you can eat more of it. Fats, saturated and

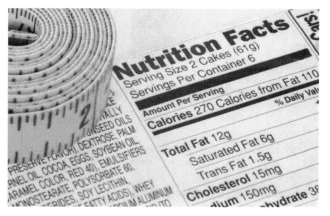

not, are still bad for weight loss. Fat portions may be extremely small but they have an extremely high calorie count. You need less fat in your daily diet than you think, and are probably already eating more of it than you realize.

Fats are a very important nutrient group. You must take in adequate essential fats or your body will not burn fat. Essential fats are very important for skin, hair and nails and many other bodily functions. Fat adds taste and usually makes you feel full and satiated. I say "usually" because most of us who are or have been overweight lack an "I'm full" switch and overeat on fat too. Diets high in fat slow down your metabolism. Why would your body burn off stored fat if you are still eating enough? Your body will let go of fat when you stop overeating it.

For the fastest weight loss I strongly suggest that you supplement with Pure Omega-3 to get your fat needs met. While a Pure Omega-3 capsule meets your dietary fat needs, I know it probably won't meet your taste needs.

I live in the real world, too. This list that follows are fats that probably will meet your taste needs but you need to eat in extreme moderation, or avoid entirely to reach your weight loss goals.

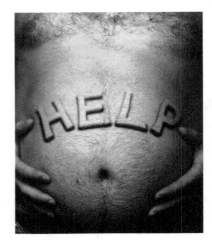

Bad fats contain larger amounts of partially-saturated, saturated, and trans fatty acids. These fats are common in processed foods such as fried foods, beef, pork, lamb, cheese, cream, butter, milk, and nut butters (both processed and unprocessed). The foods that contain fat (including "health" foods) may shock you. Maybe you've been eating them all along and wondering why you are not losing weight.

The list of "healthy" fats includes avocados, nuts, and oils—both in supplements as well as cooking oils. Use them sparingly. Don't fall into the temptation of thinking that just because they appear on a "healthy" list that you can't overdo the amount you consume, because you certainly can. Don't be one of those who eat a whole half-gallon of low fat or reduced fat ice cream just because it's "healthy". This is simply a marketing ploy and will derail your weight and fat loss efforts in a hurry. Not to mention the mental discouragement it gives. Always read labels and check for amount of grams of fat.

Nevertheless, the *right* amount of good fat is a good thing for metabolism. They contain the essential fatty acids (like fish oil) that your body cannot make on its own and play

---

FATTENING FATS

It's super important to avoid the bad fats or any fat that you can't measure or control the amount you eat. Consume too much, even if it's a good fat and you won't lose weight. Just about all processed foods (i.e., foods that God didn't make) are high in bad fats and should be avoided for fast weight loss.

Luncheon Meats	Ice Cream
Ground Meats	Margarine
Any and all Red Meats including pork,	Mayonnaise
lamb, and beef	Nondairy and Dairy Creamers
Butter	Nuts and Nut Butters
Cheeses (ALL)	Omega-3 supplements (store bought
Chips	may contain saturated fats—check
Cookies, Muffins	labels carefully)
Egg yolks	Salad Dressings
Fries	Sour Cream
Granola	Yogurts

Almost all of the protein bars and protein shakes contain fats that stop fat loss except LynFit and that's why I can only recommend LynFit products because they are best for weight loss.

---

a vital role in virtually every body function. You want these oils to be as pure as possible and you must measure them carefully. More is definitely not better. You can periodically include oils such as olive oil or a very small handful of nuts (1 ounce in a serving—be sure to measure) once daily. This is where a small slice of avocado works if you crave it.

I recommend only one tablespoon per day earlier in the day so your body has time to use it rather than store it when your metabolism naturally slows down at night to prepare for sleep. Do not consume any other fats. No butter, cream, whole milk, nor red meat. They are non-essential. Not needed. They will only do your body harm and stop the whole fat loss process. Be sure to monitor portion size (measure it out) because even essential fats can and will be stored. For fast fat loss, supplement with Pure Omega-3 to give your body what it needs, not more.

CAUTION: PROCEED WITH EXTREME PORTION CONTROL

Almonds (6)	Mackerel, salmon, sardines (1/2 cup)
Avocado (half a small one)	Olive Oil
Borage Oil	Olives
Canola Oil	Rice Bran Oil
Cooking Sprays (all)	Sesame Oil
Evening of Primrose	Sunflower Oil
Flaxseed Oil	Sunflower Seeds (1 Tablespoon)
Flaxseeds (1 Tablespoon)	

Note: All nuts and fatty fish also contain essential fats but their serving size is small and deceptive so it critical to be aware of what the serving size is. Always look for pure unprocessed oils such as "cold pressed" as processing (this includes cooking oils) destroys its benefits. Fat is 9 calories a gram, so they add up fast.

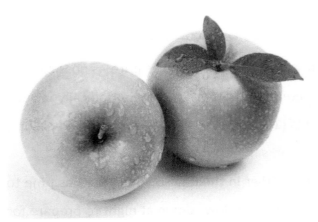

FRUIT: TOO MUCH OF A GOOD THING?

Fruit is one of the easiest snacks and desserts to transport. And while delicious, it is critical that you understand that it's not "free" like vegetables under *The Metabolism Solution*. Fruit contains sugar, and even though it's natural, it still has an effect on blood sugar. When it comes to boosting metabolism sugar is sugar. It doesn't really matter where it comes from. Fruit does contain fiber that helps slow absorption, keeps you feeling full, and contains nutrients your body needs, nevertheless, vegetables beat fruit for fat loss.

Fruit converts to sugar very quickly during digestion. This not only stops the fat-burning process but helps your body store fat. Like with fats, try to consume fruit early in the day (never past 3pm). Grapefruits and apples (especially Granny Smith) are fairly low on the glycemic index. Also, berries (strawberries, blueberries, blackberries, and raspberries) are low in sugar and higher in fiber than other fruits. Limit melons, mangoes, and pineapples. (There was once a diet fad that encouraged you to eat mostly pineapples. It didn't last.) These are very high in sugar and are probably best avoided if you cannot portion control. However, it is always better to over-eat on fruit than cookies, brownies, potato chips, or other junk food. Just keep this information in mind while trying to lose body fat.

> FRUIT HAS **STOPPED** MORE PEOPLE FROM LOSING WEIGHT THAN I CAN COUNT. CHOOSE WISELY AND USE PORTION CONTROL.

Keep your fruit to one to two servings a day. I always suggest a green apple for a 3pm snack. Be sure to measure out the amount you eat. Too much may be the culprit in your inability to lose weight. Ask any diabetic and they will tell you how their blood sugar rises from fruit.

YOUR SUGAR FIX: LOW-SUGAR FRUITS

Fruit, high in enzymes and minerals, is nature's natural cleanser. Enjoy two fruits per day maximum. Portion is 1/2 cup or as noted. Fresh or frozen (without added sugar) is fine. Always go for organic.

Apple (Granny Smith is best)	Raspberries 1 Cup
Berries (Blueberries, Blackberries) 1 cup	Strawberries 1 cup
	Oranges 1small
Cantaloupe and ALL Melons 1/2 cup	Nectarines 1 small
Grapefruit 1/2 small or 1/2 cup	Peaches 1 small
Kiwi 1 small	Pears 1 small
Cherries 10 large	Plums 2 medium

DAIRY, THE WANNABE PROTEIN

Milk-based protein is an inferior source of protein and does not possess the same metabolic-boosting properties whey protein has. Milk is high in sugar and lactose, which, of course, is not good for weight loss and can cause digestive issues. Often the calcium contained is minimal. Most commercially bought shakes and all protein bars are made from milk-based proteins—that's how they keep their prices so low. Regardless of what the label or commercial tells you, dairy will not keep you tight and lean. I have met and helped so many people who are doing so

> NONDAIRY CREAMERS (low-fat and nonfat too) are your enemies when it comes to boosting your metabolism. Don't let that "little bit" fool you. Drink your coffee black or add a little bit of your protein shake and watch the pounds fall off quickly.

much right except for the fact that they eat dairy daily and cannot understand why they are not losing weight. The low-fat yogurt you favor may have protein, but it's not whey and it's usually full of sugar, too. My clients who are fitness models and bodybuilders will not eat any dairy at all for a year before a show to really lean out. Foregoing dairy gets their skin thin and tight, and this allows you to see the fine-tuned musculature on their bodies.

That being said, this is the real world and you do need variety. I like to think of this food group, dairy, as dessert. I don't count it toward my total of protein for the day but eat it

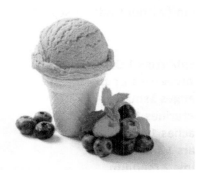

as a dessert in addition to it. I have a small child's cone of frozen yogurt everyday as a treat (I told you I wasn't perfect). This trick has kept me on track for over 20 years because I know I *can* have it daily and it satisfies me as dairy takes a long time to digest and keeps me feeling full. Keep in mind, I've already had a Complete Protein Shake to boost my metabolism—this is simply

dessert. If I am having a slow day and not eating enough protein, I will add one scoop of the shake to my yogurt to guarantee that my very slow metabolism gets what it needs.

DAIRY IS FOR COWS AND KIDS—NOT FAT LOSS

Nonfat Cheese 1 ounce (vegetable-based preferred)
Nonfat Cottage Cheese 1/2 cup
Nonfat Ricotta Cheese 1/2 cup
Nonfat/No-Sugar Yogurt, fresh or frozen, 1/2 cup
Parmesan Cheese 1 Tablespoon (sparingly, as a condiment)

Skim Milk 1 cup
*Coconut Milk 1/2 cup
*Rice Milk/Plain unsweetened 1/2 cup
*Soy Milk/Plain unsweetened 1/2 cup

*These "milks" aren't even milk-based. They are better for weight gain than loss. Remove them from your diet and see for yourself.

The dairy listed above should be used sparingly if at all until you reach your goal weight. At that time you can add a little bit back to your diet. I recommend adding one very small serving at a time and keeping a close eye on the scale to see if you gain weight—you'll know why. Note that soy and rice milk are simply not a good source of protein because they are missing amino acids and are not a complete protein like whey.

THERMOGENIC CONDIMENTS & SEASONINGS

No fats, no sauces, no cheeses. I can hear the groans. There are tasty replacements for these extras that cause you to gain weight that can imbibe your lean proteins and vegetables with mouth-watering flavors. It's true, when you cut the fat, you

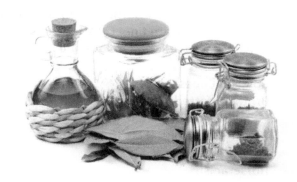

tend to cut lots of flavor, too. Learning how to season your food without relying on fats is easy. You *can* add lots of flavor without the calories. Every *lean* kitchen must have low-calorie, low-fat (with minimum sodium) seasoning staples.

Try to avoid soy, a metabolism-slowing ingredient that is in just about every marinade on a store shelf. Look for organic, gluten-free, and as little sodium as possible when buying broth. It can often be substituted in place of an oil, say in a homemade salad dressing. Aromatics such as scallions, onions, ginger, garlic, and lemongrass all fall into this group. The name tells you everything you need to know and they add that wow effect to your foods by making them not just smell good but also taste good.

COOKING WITH FLAVOR, NOT FAT

Herbs not only make food taste good, most of them are loaded with nutrients and help stimulate fat burning and detoxify your body as well. Enjoy them chopped fresh or dried.

Anise	Chives	Coriander	Fennel
Bay Leaves	Cilantro	Cumin	Garlic
Black Pepper	Cinnamon	Dill	Ginger
Cayenne	Cloves	Dried Mustard	
Parsley	Tarragon	Turmeric	

Broth can replace oil in many recipes. Tomatoes, chopped, crushed, or in a salsa add great flavor to many foods. And try to avoid salt by using salt replacements like NoSalt or Cardia. Otherwise I like to use Himalayan or Sea Salt sparingly. Canned Tomatoes, Tomato Paste, Marinara Sauce are fine. Look for the lowest sodium and fat. I love crushed tomatoes that already have garlic and onions and basil for a fast topping over fish or vegetables.

Bouillon Cubes	**Mustards (All)**
Broth, Defatted or non-fat chicken and vegetable	**Nonstick Cooking Sprays (Canola and/or Olive Oil)**
Butter Flavorings (like Butter Buds or non-fat sprays	**Salsa (2 Tablespoons look for no-fat and no-sugar and as low-carb as you can find)**
Horseradish	**Vinegars (All)**
Hot Sauce (all varieties)	
Lemon/Lime juice fresh or other	

Many spices not only add flavor but have health benefits as well. Cinnamon may help regulate blood sugar, while turmeric can help you burn fat since its main component is curcumin, which is a key ingredient in my Recovery Agent. And don't forget about metabolic-boosting cayenne. Its main ingredient, capsaicin suppresses your appetite and helps burn fat.

THERMOGENIC EATING ON THE ROAD

When you let someone else count your calories for you, you're playing a potentially dangerous game with your weight loss. Sugars and fats—and non-vegetable carbs—always find their way into your food where you least expect it. Someone's low-calorie hors d'oeuvre can be your diet saboteur. The best way to take control of your food is to make it yourself. The less you eat out, the more weight you'll lose.

Of course, you're not doomed to never eat out again. Special occasions arise, trips come up, things happen. You *can* eat out leanly if you know what to select from the menu. The best restaurant to visit is one that makes eating lean easy and without temptation. Diners and steakhouses are the establishments of choice because they often have a wide variety of items that fall on the food lists included here. My favorites? I like to order an egg white and veggie omelet at a diner with a side salad. At a steakhouse I go for salmon and a salad. Even at an airport or highway rest stop you can avoid the quick carbs. I've found sandwich shops like Subway to be fast, delicious, very economical, and metabolism-friendly—as long as I hold off on the bread.

If you're struggling to stay on track with your weight loss, it may be best to eat home until you feel strong enough to make wise choices. Once you've reached your goal, the key is learning how to plan for the splurge and make up for it afterwards. But for now, here are some tips to keep your meal thermogenic away from home.

FAST FOOD *these days offers healthier options. You can eat there if you absolutely need to. Your best bet? Order one or even two salads—if you are hungry—and your favorite burger or sandwich without the bun (or throw away the bun) and make yourself a big salad with plenty of protein from your sandwich.*

Be warned, however, just because various salads are on the menu doesn't mean it's good for weight loss if it's filled with all kinds of toppings and dressing. Always choose the lowest fat dressing available and only use as little as possible, toss the rest. If you are still hungry? Look for steamed veggies and clear broth.

Go for grilled chicken or fish and avoid fried anything at all costs. (And who can have just one crispy, salty fry?)

If the salad won't do, go with the sandwich of choice but no bun and absolutely no mayo or special sauce of any kind. Hold off on the cheese and resist the fries.

ITALIAN FOOD *is my absolute favorite. Most people turn here for pasta and pizza; unfortunately, neither is good for weight loss. These carb-heavy foods are surefire ways to stop weight loss dead in its tracks.*

Always go for fish or chicken entrees—in that order of preference. Request the veggies to be steamed with any sauce on the side. Keep the sauce on the side for your entrée too. Try a small side of tomato sauce and put two tablespoons on your main meal. You will get the Italian taste that you want; it's a good little trick and it does work for fulfilling a craving. And if you can keep that bread basket out of arm's reach you can make your favorite Italian place into a healthy restaurant. The bread isn't worth it anyway.

CHINESE FOOD *is very deceiving. It's so good and fattening—unless you know these rules. First, no hibachi for you. Anything you want on the menu must be steamed. No fried foods. My favorite is steamed shrimp with broccoli. Ask for whatever sauce comes with your dish on the side and only use two tablespoons of it. There's no deprivation because you still get the taste you want without your meal drowning in sauce and you keep control over your portion and, thus, your weight loss. If the sauce is too tempting, take your two tablespoons and have the waitperson take the rest away to avoid any extra dipping. And as with fast food, stay away from the carbs and fried food. No stir-fry, white rice, or fried rice. Goes double for the egg roll.*

MEXICAN FOOD *is another personal favorite. Don't let the waiter put any tortilla chips on your table, instead ask for an order of cut up veggies (the ones used in fajitas are my personal favorite) and dip them into the salsa. The veggies satisfy the crunch and dip cravings. And while making your menu selections, remember: No refried beans (or any beans), no sour cream, no guacamole, no flour tortillas, and no crispy taco shells. What else is there? Fajitas. They are a perfect weight-loss choice since the meat is grilled and veggies are included. Be sure to ask that they be prepared without butter. Burritos and tacos are fine—as long as you only eat only the fillings. (Remember: Avoid sour cream, guacamole, etc.) I like to order three or four shrimp and chicken tacos and then combine all the insides to create a big mish-mash of a salad. It's an instant "taco" salad without anything crunchy, except for the lettuce. No salad dressing required in a Mexican restaurant, that's what salsa is for.*

STATISTICS SHOW THAT YOU ARE **GUARANTEED** TO HAVE A WEIGHT PROBLEM IF YOU EAT OUT MORE THAN ONE MEAL A WEEK. HOW YOU CAN AVOID THE WEIGHT GAIN?

1. **BOOST YOUR METABOLISM.** Drink a shake for two meals before and after you eat out to offset the calories, balance your sugar levels, and boost your metabolism.
2. **BLOCK CARBS AND KILL CRAVINGS.** Take LynFit Carb Edge 30 minutes before your meal to block carbohydrates from being absorbed. Studies have shown that white kidney bean extract, found in Carb Edge, blocks up to 65 percent of unwanted carbs from being broken down and stored as fat.
3. **DRINK AT LEAST TWO LARGE GLASSES OF WATER BEFORE YOUR MEAL.** Do not indulge in alcohol. Try a cup of hot tea to fill you up, not out. At a party? Have some ginger ale in a champagne glass.
4. **KNOW BEFORE YOU GO.** Check the menu online or call ahead before you select a restaurant to avoid getting stuck with fat-inducing choices. Choose what you'll eat before you get there. Many restaurants also offer a "light" menu. Select from it and you can save 800 or more calories.
5. **EAT YOUR VEGETABLES.** All 10 servings. Focus on eating steamed veggies with sauces on the side—and ask that they be prepared without butter.
6. **SLIM DOWN YOUR SALAD AND EAT AS MUCH AS YOU CAN.** You'll be fuller by the time the entrée is served and avoid temptations. To keep your salad lean say yes to vegetables but "no" to avocado, cheese, beans, croutons, raisins (all dried fruit), bacon, yolks, and nuts. Pick a vinaigrette over a creamy dressing option. Or try my secret dressing: mustard mixed with vinegar. Top it all off with shrimp or salmon. You can save up to 800 calories.
7. **SHARING IS CARING.** Split an entree with your dinner companion or ask the waiter to wrap up half of it to bring home and save for tomorrow. You'll save calories and money.
8. **FILL UP WITH BROTH.** Broth-based soups like chicken noodle—without the noodles—minestrone, garden vegetable, and miso save hundreds of calories and keep you full and satisfied.

DRINK MORE WATER, BOOST YOUR METABOLISM 3%

Did you know that 9 times out of 10 when you think your body is sending you hunger signals they're really thirst signals? Dehydration can slow your metabolism by three percent. Getting enough water helps your body cleanse itself and flush out waste. It is imperative to drink half your weight in ounces of water daily. That may sound like a lot, but it's not that bad. Weigh 150 pounds? That's 75 ounces of water, which is about 4 1/2 standard-sized (16.9 OZ) water bottles a day.

> **DEHYDRATION SLOWS YOUR METABOLISM BY 3 PERCENT. DRINK *HALF* YOUR BODY WEIGHT IN OUNCES OF WATER DAILY FOR OPTIMUM HYDRATION.**

For some of you that may be easy, for me—not so much. I need a little motivation when it comes to drinking water. I love pure, ice-cold water when I'm working out, but at other times, especially if the weather is neither too hot nor too cold, I add calorie-free, fat-free flavor to entice my taste buds to reach for a bottle of water. I also leave visual cues to get myself to drink. An eye-catching pitcher of water left on a counter

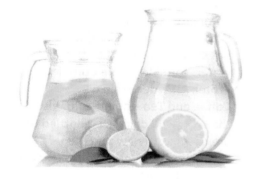

alongside a pretty glass reminds me to stop and drink every time I walk by. I love to add cucumber slices with ginger or lemon slices to my pitcher. I've even been known to try and float the occasional melon ball or two.

I've been asked many times about the sugar-free packets made to add to bottled water. While not ideal,

> **WHAT ABOUT DIET SODA?** It is better to kill a craving once in a while with a can of diet soda (and they can really hit the spot) than it is to eat 300 calories trying to avoid diet (0 calorie) soda. You don't have to be too rigid. Your body will begin to crave clean, pure water the more you drink it. It takes time, so be patient and don't worry if you need to wean yourself off high-sugar sodas and juices in the beginning. Sometimes a diet soda is just what you need to keep you satisfied and on track.

TRY THESE THIRST-QUENCHING, DELICIOUS, AND HYDRATING TRICKS TO ENCOURAGE YOU TO DRINK MORE WATER

1. **Water with lemon or lime. It's light and fresh.**
2. **Add cinnamon to create a slimming water.**
3. **Try cucumbers and ginger for an irresistible fresh, clean treat.**
4. **Water with floating fruit. Take whatever citrus, berries, apples, nectarines—you name it—lying around, slice them up, and float them in large pitcher. Kids will love the juicy fruit when the water is gone.**
5. **Skinny Hot Chocolate. My personal favorite. Mix 1 scoop of Chocolate Complete Protein powder with water. Warm it up (do not boil) for a skinny hot chocolate treat. For chocolate water, sprinkle a little Complete Protein powder in ice water.**
6. **Coffee and Tea—hot or cold. Just hold the sugar and dairy. Diet bottled teas are okay every now and then.**
7. **Zero-calorie flavored waters. Packets or already bottled.**
8. **Sparkling waters (carbonated waters as well as mineral waters) such as Perrier and Pellegrino, seltzers (flavored and plain), and Club soda. Try a splash (and I mean a quick splash—not a glass) of juice in your seltzer as you wean yourself from sugary drinks.**
9. **Make flavored ice cubes using any of the above calorie-free drinks and add them to your water.**
10. **Coffee water. Burns fats faster than water alone. Add a splash of coffee.**

they work in a pinch. I keep the little packets of Crystal Light Ice Peach Tea and Lemonade in my purse and at my home to add to water when I'm desperate and haven't been drinking like I should.

These packets help promote water drinking, and drinking water always keeps you from over-eating. Drink at least two large glasses of water before your meals and you can lose an average of 16 pounds in 3 months.

Remember: Much of the time when you think you're hungry, you are actually thirsty. Before you reach for something to chew, try a drink first. These are my favorite calorie-free beverages (and they count toward your ounces of water) that keep me—and will keep you—satisfied and feeling full. They hit the spot without adding any extra calories. Try them, warm or hot, just don't add a drop of dairy.

THE LEGAL SNACK ATTACK

It happens to me, too. I have those moments where I just can't help myself. Sometimes, you just need to eat, even when you know you shouldn't. There *are* foods that are helpful to have on hand for such binge moments. But remember Rule #1 when it comes to foods you can and cannot eat: When in doubt, don't! Stay away from foods you can't binge on—it'll slow your weight loss, you'll have too much guilt, and it won't be worth it. Before you start that binge ask yourself what you're *really* feeling. Are you sad? Angry? Bored? Lonely? Tired? Food won't

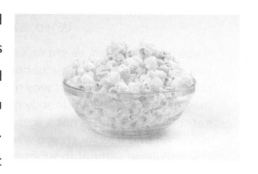

fix it, but only make it worse. Avoid eating whenever and wherever possible. Food is the problem, not the solution. And if it's been more than three hours since you last ate, it's time eat.

If snack you must, choose foods with the lowest caloric content like those on the list below. I'll be honest, when I'm truly craving, it's for something I want to nosh a lot of, not simply "snack." That's why this list is made up of high-volume low-calorie foods that won't have you going over your calorie budget when you have more than just one. Always make sure that you have eaten all of the vegetables that you were supposed to if you're still looking for more

IF YOU CANNOT PORTION CONTROL IT, DON'T EAT IT!

food, it just might be because you didn't get your 10 vegetables in. And if you've tried everything on the list, and still feel that yen, there's always another Complete Protein Shake made with water. Blend it in a blender for 1 to 2 minutes to add air—the air will make you feel full.

GOT SNACKS?

Air-Popped Popcorn, 3 cups (60 calories)
Clear Broth Soup
Fudgsicles (25 to 40 calories)
Garden Salad
Green Apple, 1 small
Sugarless gum

Sugar-Free Candy, 2 pieces
Sugar Free Gelatin
Sugar-Free Popsicles (15 to 25 calories)
Tomato Juice
Tootsie Roll Pop (25 calories)

WHO SAID CHEATERS NEVER LOSE?

If you are stuck on a weight loss plateau or you need to lose that last stubborn 5 to 10 pounds, cheating *the right way* on your diet may be exactly what your body needs. Don't get too excited, this is not a license to eat whatever and how much you want. Overindulging without forethought can take up to a solid week of clean eating to get back on track.

The secret to cheating without gaining an ounce is to prepare your metabolism ahead of time—boost your metabolism before you indulge so that when you do cheat, your body is ready to torch those calories instead of storing them. Boosting your metabolism and then cheating sends your metabolic fire into a fireball mode. That metabolic bonfire will power you through that plateau and blast off that extra 5 to 10 pounds.

What makes planned cheating different? *You control the cheat*; it doesn't control you. When a cheat controls you it's a binge, and binging slows weight loss, sometimes considerably.

Have a special dinner occasion coming up? You can block weight gain by planning when you will cheat so you can prepare your body for it. First, power up your metabolism with protein and vegetables—not carbs. I cannot stress it enough; protein is *the* necessary ingredient to boost your metabolism. Wake up to a Complete Protein Shake and then keep it "no carb" throughout the day. Don't even add fruit. This way, you save your carbs for dinner. And don't forget a Carb Edge before you go out to block those carbohydrates from being stored as fat.

When all else fails try to tame the beast by eating yummy things that are high in nutrients to help fat loss and not cause it. Hint: They are green.

Don't worry if you fall off the wagon. You are human and it's expected because no one is perfect. Eighty percent perfect is as good as you'll get, even when it comes to staying on your weight-loss plan. Let it go and get right back on. Fix a binge in one day by going back to the 48-Hour Metabolic Cleanse. It can boost your metabolism. Boost your metabolism and fix your worst eating day.

MY FAVORITE GUILT-FREE INDULGENCES

COOKIES AND CREAM "ICE CREAM" SHAKE:
- 2 TSP of Cookies and Cream pudding mix
- 2 scoops of Chocolate Complete Protein Shake
- 1/2 cup water
- 5 Ice cubes

Blend together for 20-30 seconds or until desired consistency is reached. Garnish with dark chocolate shavings.

TOFFEE AND APPLE BITES: Slice up your favorite apple and place Lean Bar pieces on top for a sweet treat.

MICROWAVE LOW CALORIE KETTLE CORN: Look for 100 calorie packs. Follow instructions and enjoy.

Rules and Numbers for Weight Loss

The most effective way to lose weight is to follow a strict, structured plan. It works faster and is ten times more effective than putting a plan together yourself. Following a plan or trying to create your own, you must stick with foods that boost your metabolism. Math is important to weight loss success. Never forget this formula for your daily calorie requirement. These numbers are critical when trying to lose weight.

> **Dieters who eat the same thing daily not only lose more weight faster but keep it off longer.**

YOUR GOAL WEIGHT X 10 = TOTAL CALORIES FOR THE DAY

So if you are reaching for 120 pounds, you need to consume 1,200 calories maximum a day to hit that goal. *The Metabolism Solution* has this already taken care of, but if you decide to try the do-it-yourself approach, here's what you need to know:

1. **Start you day with whey to boost your metabolism by 25 percent.** Within one hour of waking, drink a Complete Protein Shake or have a Lean Bar when portability is needed.
2. **Limit fat.** Keep your daily fat intake to 15 grams max for women and 20 grams maximum for men and teens. Choose only essential fats.
3. **Be careful with carbs.** Consume carbohydrates (if you insist on eating them), before 3pm If you're losing too slowly, drop carbs completely. (vegetables do not count)
4. **Power your metabolism with protein.** 25 grams of lean protein (see list) per meal.
5. **Read labels to be lean.** Check calorie counts and weight and measure everything or look it up in a calorie book. This one simple step can make or break your weight loss.
6. **Water for weight loss.** Drink half your body weight in ounces of water daily. That's 8 to 10 glasses a day—minimum.
7. **Snack slim.** Keep snacks at 100 calories or less. Better yet, go for veggies or fruit.

8. **Timing is everything.** Keep a minimum of three hours between meals. If you eat in between, your body cannot digest the food and will store it as fat. This could also cause insulin to rise and slow down all the metabolic boosting you've been working so hard on.

9. **Food is only half your day.** Eat all your meals in a 12-hour window: 7am to 7pm.

10. **Get HUNGRY!** Hunger is a good sign. It means your body is about to burn fat. The feeling will dissipate. You don't need to instantly gratify every food craving. Find another way to entertain yourself—change a thought and move muscle, anything BUT succumb to eating again. You will not be literally starving. It was a pivotal moment for me when I learned it was okay to be hungry. Hunger is a sign your body is about to start burning fat. Don't let it scare you.

IF YOU BITE IT, WRITE IT!

In my 25 years I have learned a lot about how food journals can be helpful. But I've also learned that most people don't use them enough and aren't always totally honest when they do. *Honest* food journals work—studies show that people who journal exactly what they ate lost more weight and kept it off. What I find helps the most is logging your bad days for true insight on you and food.

If you bite, chew, sip, or chug it, write it down. What you eat in private shows up on the scale (or your body), so be honest with yourself. Be sure to add what you put on your food or in your coffee, as it's these small things that often add up and cause us to gain weight in the first place. List how much of each food you eat, the time of day, and how you felt when you ate it. Did you eat standing up in front of the refrigerator? Or were you sitting down eating slowly in a relaxed state? All this matters. Rate your hunger on a scale from 1 to 5 with 5 being the most hungry (real hunger, not head hunger) and list that too. After all, most of the eating we do isn't real hunger at all but rather stress showing up in our food.

> IF YOU BITE IT, WRITE IT! EVERY MORSEL OF IT. THE GOOD DAYS AREN'T NECESSARY, LOG THE REALLY BAD ONES FOR BEST INSIGHT.

LynFit Nutrition Metabolic Boosting Food Journal

Use this check list to help you stay on track every day. Be sure to write down everything you eat each day and mark off the corresponding box. The number of boxes shown for each food group is the number of servings to be eaten each day. If you notice several blank boxes, focus in eating foods from the missing groups to BOOST your metabolism! Don't forget to check off your exercise and supplement boxes!

	SUNDAY	MONDAY	TUESDAY	WEDNESDAY	THURSDAY	FRIDAY	SATURDAY	SUNDAY
Water	⚪⚪⚪⚪⚪⚪⚪⚪	⚪⚪⚪⚪⚪⚪⚪⚪	⚪⚪⚪⚪⚪⚪⚪⚪	⚪⚪⚪⚪⚪⚪⚪⚪	⚪⚪⚪⚪⚪⚪⚪⚪	⚪⚪⚪⚪⚪⚪⚪⚪	⚪⚪⚪⚪⚪⚪⚪⚪	⚪⚪⚪⚪⚪⚪⚪⚪
Protein Shake/Lean Bar	⚪⚪	⚪⚪	⚪⚪	⚪⚪	⚪⚪	⚪⚪	⚪⚪	⚪⚪
Vegetables	⚪⚪⚪⚪⚪⚪⚪⚪	⚪⚪⚪⚪⚪⚪⚪⚪	⚪⚪⚪⚪⚪⚪⚪⚪	⚪⚪⚪⚪⚪⚪⚪⚪	⚪⚪⚪⚪⚪⚪⚪⚪	⚪⚪⚪⚪⚪⚪⚪⚪	⚪⚪⚪⚪⚪⚪⚪⚪	⚪⚪⚪⚪⚪⚪⚪⚪
Fish/Protein	⚪	⚪	⚪	⚪	⚪	⚪	⚪	⚪
Fruit	⚪	⚪	⚪	⚪	⚪	⚪	⚪	⚪
Snack	⚪	⚪	⚪	⚪	⚪	⚪	⚪	⚪
Supplements/AM	⚪	⚪	⚪	⚪	⚪	⚪	⚪	⚪
Supplements/PM	⚪	⚪	⚪	⚪	⚪	⚪	⚪	
Sleep (list hours)								WORSHIP!
Pray/Meditate (check)								
Cardio (list length)								
Metabolic Workouts #								
Body Weight/BMI								

Lean Proteins
LynFit Protein Shake
egg whites - 3
all fish - 4oz.
turkey - 3oz.
chicken breast - 3oz.
LynFit Lean Bar

Veggies
all lettuce - 3 cups
spinach - 1/2 cup
all green veggies - 1/2 cup
cabbage - 1 cup
broccoli
string beans
brussel sprouts
zucchini
yellow squash

Low Sugar Fruits
apple - 1 small
blueberries - 1/2 cup
raspberries - 1/2 cup
grapefruit - 1/2 cup

Calorie Free Beverages
water
green tea
black coffee
calorie-free seltzer

Snacks
LynFit lean bar
cut up veggies
complete protein shake
sugar-free, fat-free Jell-O
15 calorie popsicles/fudgesicles
3 cups air-popped popcorn
pudding cups < 100 calories
100 calorie popcorn
(6) almonds < 100 calories
yogurt < 100 calories
Tic Tacs

Supplements For Fat Loss
LynFit Complete Protein Shake
LynFit Lean Bar
LynFit Cutting Edge
LynFit Carb Edge
LynFit Raspberry Ketone Cleanse
LynFit Lean Sleep
LynFit Pure Omega-3
LynFit Daily Power Shot (if needed)
LynFit Recovery Agent (if needed)

Visit LynFit.com today for more metabolic boosting information

Researchers from the Fred Hutchinson Cancer Research Center found that dieters who kept food journals lost six pounds more than those who didn't journal. And that's not even the best part. Food journals have proven to be more helpful than simply serving as a list keeping track of what you eat. They keep you accountable for what you put in your mouth and they tip off your emotional triggers cause you to overeat. Food journaling reveals if you skip meals, eat out often, or lack pre-meal planning, behaviors which can lead to overeating. Once revealed, these behaviors can be addressed. It's also critical to journal where you are while you are eating and your feelings at that moment. Were you out with friends? Alone? Upset over a disagreement with a friend? These kinds of things very much affect weight loss if you respond to them with food. After much research, I use the food journal shown above with my clients. (You can download it from my website lynfit.com.) It lets you check off supplements. While it is extremely helpful and useful for keeping track of what you eat, it only works if you're honest. That's why I'm now asking you to track your bad days. From those days especially, you can learn what needs to be changed with how you eat. Remember, what you eat accounts for 80 percent, if not more, in your battle to lose weight. Take a moment, and enter your food intake in a journal. Be sure to write what you were feeling *before* you ate as well as what you craved. That will help you troubleshoot next time. Journals aren't about creating more work, they are a way to track so you can look back and see where you went off.

THE DIET DIAGNOSER

The fastest way to figure out where you are off so that you know exactly what you need to do to lose weight today.

1) Did you drink a Complete Protein Shake at least once without adding fruit or dairy?
2) Did you eat vegetables? Greens or high-sugar types like carrots and tomatoes?
3) Did you drink 10 glasses of water?
4) Did you eat carbs? (Be on carb alert. They show up everywhere, check all your labels.)
5) Did you "slip up" on any of the following diet destroyers:
   - Cheese
   - Milk (Soy or Other)
   - Oils
   - Nuts
   - Red Meat
   - Alcohol
   - Candy or Cookies
   - Pasta
   - Bread
   - Excess Fruit
6) Have you weighed and measured everything?
7) Did you forget to take your Cutting Edge, Carb Edge, or whatever supplement your metabolism requires for weight loss?
8) Did you walk every day for 45 minutes to an hour?
9) Did you do the Metabolic Boosting Workouts (page 163)? They're "medicine" for your metabolism.
10) Are you worried that you won't lose weight and are so stressed that it's affecting your weight loss?

The Metabolism Solution works every time when you follow it. Everyone loses weight. No one fails. So if the scale is stuck, it's time to slip out of diet denial and keep re-assessing what you're eating until you find the weight gain culprit. It took me years to figure this out. The truth was I didn't want to admit or accept that the "little bit" of raisins or milk or my once-a-week breakfast of oatmeal could do so much harm. Once I decided to stop eating these foods, the scale dropped right away. You have to challenge yourself—step out of your comfort zone—if you are serious about boosting your metabolism so you lose weight faster.

WAIT, DON'T REACH FOR THAT DOUGHNUT

Bumps on the road to weight loss show up in a food journal. A journal helps diagnose the behavior underneath your overeating. Once you get to the behavior underneath, the problem (overeating) takes care of itself. Here are some tips on avoiding these obstacles.

- Bored? Tackle an item on your to-do list.
- Lonely? Call a friend.
- Poor planning? Make a plan or plan to fail.
- Angry? Exercise instead.
- Craving crunch? Popcorn or veggies satisfy that need.
- Craving comfort? Make a cup of Skinny Hot Chocolate.
- Tired? Take a nap or go to bed earlier.
- At a restaurant? Plan what you will eat ahead of time.
- Hungry off meal times? Drink a glass of water and journal instead.

CLEANSE, BOOST, REPEAT

The goal is to not only eat healthy (as eating from the lists of foods on the preceding pages will have you do) but to lose weight. So, to jumpstart your metabolism, you need to re-boot it. That's where the Cleanse comes in. Your average cleanse—and there are many to choose from on the market—purports to detoxify and heal your body mostly by eliminating waste and not necessarily nourishing the rest of you. Detoxifying is important. It helps make it easier for your body to burn calories, but detoxifying the *wrong* way will damage your metabolism and make weight loss even more difficult.

Juicing has been popular for years now, but it's not a good plan to follow for weight loss. While you might lose a pound or two because you're only drinking and not eating for a day or more, juiced vegetables and fruits will jackhammer your blood sugar through the roof. And are you going to be able to keep that pound off and build on it? You can juice to your heart's content, but you will not find a faster or better way to boost your metabolism than the Metabolic Boosting Cleanse. The best part? You get to eat, not just drink. Eating and chewing your food (and especially your vegetables) is always best because then you're burning calories during digestion. Juicing breaks down food into such small particles that are digested very quickly, not requiring as many calories for the process. And when food digests so quickly, your blood sugar spikes, and this causes your body to store fat, specifically around the midsection, hips, and thighs. I call this "the insulin band" and if you "wear" such a band, it's proof positive that you're eating too many of the wrong carbohydrates and sugars.

It's called a "cleanse" because it alkalinizes your body, returning it to its proper PH levels (sweets, meats, and processed foods create acidity), detoxifies, and re-boots your metabolism, but it is so much more. This is the important first step on the road to weight loss following *The Metabolism Solution*. The Metabolic Boosting Cleanse is the fastest, safest cleanse on the market and, the best part is, it's so safe you can repeat it as often as needed. In fact, some of my clients feel so much better on it that they follow the Cleanse and live on

> **HOW DO YOU KNOW** if you need to cleanse? Here are the telltale signs that your body is begging for one:
>
> - **Cravings**
> - **Bloating, feeling heavy, constipated**
> - **Hard time losing weight.**
> - **Depression, moodiness**
> - **Tired, lacking energy**
> - **Muscle aches and pains**
> - **Sleep problems**
> - **Skin eruptions/eczema**
> - **Sick, frequent colds/headaches**
> - **Sinus and allergy problems**

it 2 to 3 days a week as a way to control their weight and gain health or feel better. Can you say that about another cleanse?

You start the Cleanse the way I recommend you start every morning; with a Complete Protein Shake. The high-quality whey protein feeds the muscle and starves the fat. You won't find high-quality protein in a juice cleanse. Lunch is the same. For a change of pace, check out my shake recipes on page 47 and for a truly metabolic-revving alternative, add some greens. You read that right. Who knew that kale, cucumber, and celery could taste so cool and refreshing in a vanilla Complete Protein Shake.

There's no snacking between meals, but you can fill up on green tea, which is full of antioxidants. Give your body time to digest, wait at least three hours between meals, and let yourself feel hungry—that's a sign your body is burning fat. Dinner consists of vegetables and a lean, clean, white protein like fish. White fish is preferred over salmon, chicken, and turkey because it is less fatty. Think green and white when it comes to food: green for vegetables and white for fish. These are the foods that meet your body's needs and boost your metabolism. And don't forget to drink plenty of water—10 glasses a day (green tea counts toward the requirement).

THE LEAN GREEN CLEANSING MACHINE

Cleansing is the best way to jump-start your fat loss when you do it right. Try this re-energizing and detoxifying shake to put you on the weight loss path. Scared you won't like the veggies in it? Start slow and try one new veggie each day. Most people love kale, cucumber, and spinach because they are so mild tasting.

- **1 cup water or black coffee (coffee is loaded with antioxidants)**
- **4 scoops of your favorite Complete Protein flavor (results are not guaranteed when using other shakes as they are loaded with inferior protein and sugar)**
- **1 large cucumber**
- **1 fistful of kale**
- **1 stalk of celery**
- **1 big broccoli stem**
- **1/2 peeled lemon**

Wash and prep ingredients. Add to blender and blend away. Makes 2 servings—your lunch shake is ready to go.

Supplements are key to the entire process: A Daily Power Shot in the morning, a Pure Omega-3 - at 3pm, two Raspberry Ketone Cleanse with dinner, and a Lean Sleep just

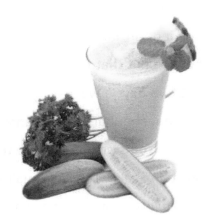

before bedtime. Sleep is where true detoxing takes place, so it's best to sleep 7 to 8 hours, and if you're anything like me, you need a little help. These help pack the Cleanse with the extra oomph needed to re-boot your metabolism.

Once you've started the re-boot of your metabolism with the Cleanse, you have completed the first steps to weight loss and can add some additional foods to your dinner and later your lunch (stick with those on the lists). Throw out all of the junk food you have laying around and prepare by going shopping and buying only what you need. Bring the food lists with you. If you need to eat out, call the restaurant ahead of time and ask them to prepare your fish and green salad without dressing, croutons, or cheese. Broil your fish with lemon juice instead of butter, oil, or any extra salt. Then sit down and write out your meals—and be exact. Write down what you will eat and when. Keep in mind; it's best to eat between the hours of 7am and 7pm and no later than 8pm.

> **THE METABOLIC-BOOSTING CLEANSE**
>
> **BREAKFAST**
> - **Complete Protein Shake**
> - **Daily Power Shot to provide nutrients and energy**
> - **Green Tea as desired throughout day**
>
> **LUNCH**
> - **Complete Protein Shake**
>
> **MID-DAY**
> - **1 Pure Omega-3 to curb cravings**
>
> **DINNER**
> - **Green vegetables (5 1/2 cup sevings) and white fish (4 oz.)**
> - **2 Raspberry Ketone Cleanse**
>
> **BEDTIME**
> - **Lean Sleep to provide restful and revitalizing sleep**

After cleansing for two or three days, you can vary your dinner and add a snack of a green apple or other legal snack as described on page 109 along with a Pure Omega-3. The Cutting Edge, Carb Edge, and Accelerator supplements can give your metabolism that extra kick if added as well. If you stick to this Metabolic-Boosting Meal Plan, you can lose up to 1 pound a day. *If* you stick with it. As you lose weight, you can add in other foods from the food lists in this chapter and take them out if they interfere with the pounds coming off. (Your journaling will let you know)

What about constipation? Staying regular is crucial during this time, but you don't want to spend your day in the bathroom either, which is how some cleanses operate. If you're eating enough veggies and drinking enough water, you will stay regular. Aim for 10 veggies per day minimum (see list page 93) and 10 glasses of water daily.

METABOLIC-BOOSTING MEAL PLAN

Exercise is important in so many ways, but it's what and how much you eat that really determines your weight loss. This is the base plan that you can stick with for the rest of your life. No one is perfect, you will sneak in foods and entire meals you shouldn't, but as long as you get back on the plan, you'll get back to losing weight and keeping it off.

Starting your day with a Complete Protein shake makes all the difference. This one drink revs up your metabolism for the rest of the day. If you just replace your usual breakfast with a protein shake, you'll see a difference, but if you follow *The Metabolism Solution*, you'll see change.

Once the weight begins to come off, you can replace your lunchtime shake with vegetables and a lean protein. You'll find plenty of satisfying and filling foods to choose from within these pages and some metabolism-revving recipes as well. If you stop losing weight or slow down, go back to a shake for lunch. Give it a try; you have nothing to lose but the pounds.

BREAKFAST
- Complete Protein shake made with water or Lean Bar
- Black coffee or tea
  - Supplements: 1 Cutting Edge, 1 Carb Edge

SNACK
- Small apple

LUNCH
- Complete Protein shake made with water or Lean Bar
  - Supplements: 1 Cutting Edge, 1 Carb Edge

SNACK
- Small apple or any fruit from List (page 99) or legal snack (page 107)
  - Supplements: 1 Pure Omega-3, 1 Carb Edge if needed

DINNER
- Choose 4 ounces of any lean protein from the list (page 87) and a large salad with a minimum of 5 vegetables from the list (page 93)

SNACK
- Anything from Legal Snack list (page 109)

BEDTIME
- Lean Sleep if needed

QUICK TIPS
- **Men and Teens:** Add 1 to 2 additional scoops of Complete Protein to your shakes or 3 to 4 egg whites. Or add an additional 1 to 2 ounces of fish to your meal plan to increase daily protein.
- **Still hungry?** Have more salad, vegetables, or clear broth; any of these will keep you satisfied and feeling full. A cup of tea or hot water with lemon works great after a meal too.
- **No alcohol or juice for the leanest results.**
- **Ideal Meal Times:** Breakfast at 7 a.m., snack at 10 a.m., lunch at 1 p.m., snack at 4 p.m., dinner at 7 p.m. No eating after 8 p.m.

Snack Options: A snack can satisfy head hunger and hold you over until your next meal. Snacks below boost your metabolism too.
- Cut-up veggies or garden salad with fat-free dressing
- Complete Protein shake or Lean Bar
- Sugar-free, fat-free Jell-O or pudding
- Sugar-free, fat-free, low-calorie popsicle or Fudgsicle
- 1 serving (under 100 calories) fat-free low-sugar frozen yogurt or ice cream
- Air popped popcorn (3 cups) or 100-calorie bag Smart Food or microwave popcorn.
- Small apple or 1/2 cup unsweetened or sugar-free applesauce (I like Muscleman's)
- Sugarless gum, menthol cough drops, Altoids, or fireballs help stop cravings
- 100-calorie serving or almonds (about 8 to 10 nuts)

If that isn't enough to keep you regular, however, I suggest taking 3 Raspberry Ketone Cleanse for two days in a row at the most convenient time for you. Most people take it at 10am or at bedtime, allowing sufficient time for it to do its job. Take Raspberry Ketone Cleanse at a time you'll remember and do not mix it with other supplements. After the initial 48 hours, continue taking 1 to 2 each day until the bottle is finished, or keep it on hand to use for those Cleanse days you'll want to do each week.

One final thing to consider while losing weight using *The Metabolism Solution* is the use of over-the-counter medication, much of which is metabolism-deadening—particularly antihistamines. If you can (and check with your doctor), consider not taking them. You may very well find you can make do without them once you detoxify and begin eating clean.

The average weight-loss program is full of don'ts. Don't eat this and don't eat that. Don't ever eat entire categories of food. I want you to enjoy food. Nevertheless, if you want to lose weight and keep it off, you have to make changes to your diet to see changes in your body. I still live to eat, and what I've come to realize is that successful weight loss

> THE GREATER THE VARIETY OF FOODS IN YOUR HOUSE, THE MORE LIKELY YOU'RE TO HAVE A WEIGHT PROBLEM. KEEP IT SIMPLE.

lies in *replacing* favorite foods with lighter, leaner versions and having a Complete Protein Shake. Use the foods found on the preceding lists to create a meal plan that suits you best. Remember that you must: 1) Drink a Complete Protein Shake for breakfast every day; 2) Drink at least 10 cups of water a day; 3) Eat 10 vegetable servings; 4) Keep 3 hours minimum and 4 hours maximum betwee meals to keep your blood sugar levels balanced; and 5) Eat right at night by choosing a 4-ounce serving of lean protein and at least 5 vegetables for dinner. For leanest results, do not drink acoholic beverages or any juice. Try to fit your meals in a 12-hour window: breakfast at 7am, lunch at 1pm and dinner at 7pm. Do not eat after 8pm.

Remember, it's always better to eat frozen vegetables than none at all and adding a lean protein to the veggies makes it a complete meal. When you are feeding a whole family dinner, I rely on the recipes in Chapter 9. It's easy to design a seven-day dinner plan that works for every one with these; I base my family meals on it.

There's something to be said for sticking to the same daily meals. Dieters who eat the same thing daily not only lose more weight faster but keep it off longer. You can take the guess work out of meal planning by creating a family meal calendar and sticking with it. Your life will be easier and you'll live leaner.

Five

WHO DECIDES THE SERVING SIZE ANYWAY?

'Ve always told people that when it comes to portion size, "Don't blame me, I don't make the rules". While writing this book I began to really wonder, who *does* decide? Who decides that one bottle will have two servings? That while the package comes with two pieces, it's only one serving? That 15 potato chips from the bag is how much you should eat at one time? Why does it seem so arbitrary sometimes? Figuring out serving sizes is a confusing issue—made more confusing by the ever-growing portion size in the United States. Can it be a coincidence that portions have grown larger every year and obesity rates have increased along with them? At an absurd rate I might add. If I may paraphrase Martha; Supersizing is *not* a good thing.

First of all, you need to know that portion and serving size are not the same thing. A portion is how much you put on your plate; a serving size is a measured specific amount of food that makes it easier for consumers to compare when buying. They are similar, but not interchangeable. Health was not considered when coming up with serving size. It was created and ordered to be on food packages in 1994 as an industry standard, not to help you make smart food choices. When it comes to portions, you're supposed to figure that one out on your own.

Because there is so much confusion over what a *true* serving size is there is no standard reference point for you to determine what the appropriate amount of food to eat is. Let alone what you should be eating in the first place. Package labels differ so much from brand to brand that you cannot assume that the same amount of low-fat potato chips, say 15 chips per serving, doesn't change from one brand to the next. Guess what? It does.

Every day I have people crying out to me in despair saying, "I have always been able to eat this food without gaining weight and now when I eat it I gain 5 pounds immediately". Or

> LABELS, APPS, AND ONLINE DIET FITNESS PLANS ARE MORE LIKELY TO SABOTAGE YOU THAN HELP YOU LOSE WEIGHT.

"I track everything I eat in XYZ app and yet I still can't lose belly fat". Trying to find the reasons for this is a little bit harder than it used to be. You may think you're eating the right way, but you really aren't. It's getting harder to teach people the "why's" behind all these dilemmas and that's because you have to pretty much unlearn what you've been taught about food portions and labels. I had to forget everything I had learned and start fresh. Only then did I begin to lose weight in spite of my slow metabolism.

Before I get further into portion size and labels, you need to first understand these five weight loss truths.

1. After age 30, everything changes metabolically—accept that you need to do things differently to lose weight.

2. Every year of your life your metabolism will slow down.

3. Whatever you think you're eating according to an app on your phone or PC is far off base. Use them as rough guides, not gospel. Did you know that these apps are allowed to be off by 20 percent in what they tell you? That's enough to stop weight loss and maybe even cause weight gain.

4. Your body only needs one-third of the food you eat every day for health and wellness. The other two-thirds is what you *want* to eat, not what you need.

5. Your belief system affects everything about your weight loss. If you don't believe something will work, you won't even try.

So what does this all have to do with serving' sizes you ask? Lots!

IT'S NOT YOUR FAULT

The most important things I can teach you is that you need to take appropriate steps (like drinking a protein shake everyday) to help offset these weight loss truths *if* you don't want to gain weight every year. Read the previous chapter, Thermogenic Eating for Radical Weight Loss, again so you know which foods to eat and stick with them. Use the serving sizes and portions I recommend. And read labels carefully. I often spend time with clients showing them how label shenanigans affect their attempts at weight loss. And don't even get me started on weight loss apps. I have yet to find one I could even recommend with reservations. They are the problem, not the solution. Eating too many calories and eating the wrong foods is what actually slows your metabolism.

Following the suggestions of labels and apps can lead you to gain weight if not stagnate. I can tell you story after story about clients who spend far too much time arguing

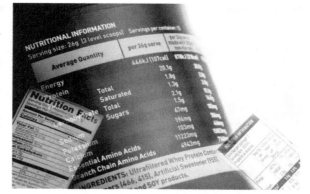

with me that that they are eating perfectly, even meticulously according to their apps or incredibly detailed computerized plans, yet still cannot lose weight or an inch of belly fat. (Now if they only spent the time they spend arguing with me walking, they would be at goal weight or maybe even need to gain a few.)

As much as it may sound like an excuse, the system really is at fault here. It's not you. Apps and labels can sabotage you. Do you know who sets the serving sizes you see on the side panel of your favorite food or on the computer diet and fitness program you use? You're going to be surprised. It's you. Well, people like you.

You might think that in this day and age labeling and servings would be designed by a more scientific approach. I always assumed that serving sizes were calculated to goals. So if you are trying to lose weight, you should eat this certain amount, but if you are trying to gain or maintain it would be a different amount. Makes perfect sense that serving sizes should be

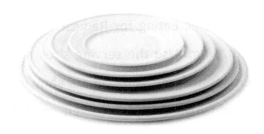

different when you're a 6-foot tall 30-year-old man and a 4-foot 9-inch woman who is 55. But how is it that growing children, teens, and people who are active are told to use the same serving sizes that you are when trying to lose weight and shrink your waistline? Have you ever thought of it this way? Shouldn't serving sizes be a little bit different if you are tall or short or whether you have lots of muscle or very little muscle? Ideally, shouldn't serving sizes factor in the rate you burn calories, take into account your metabolism's speed?

I speak from my personal experience and the experiences of all the people I have helped over the years. Every time I tried to follow the food pyramid recommendations put forth by the U.S. government—and by the way, I was meticulous about serving sizes—I still gained weight. My metabolism is so slow that if I even look at 1/2 a serving of pasta I gain 5 pounds, yet my 6-foot tall and fairly active husband skips pasta at one meal and loses 10 pounds. (Okay, so that's a *little* bit of an exaggeration, but it sure feels like it.) I'm hoping this gets you thinking. You really have to be your own detective when it comes to losing weight.

> SHOULDN'T SERVING SIZES BE A LITTLE DIFFERENT IF YOU ARE TALL OR SHORT OR WHETHER YOU HAVE LOTS OF MUSCLE OR VERY LITTLE MUSCLE? IDEALLY, SHOULDN'T SERVING SIZES FACTOR IN THE RATE YOU BURN CALORIES AND TAKE INTO ACCOUNT YOUR METABOLISM'S SPEED?

Serving guidelines cannot serve as gospel, but merely as a rough gauge. The scale will show you every time if you're on the right track. If the scale isn't moving, you're still eating too much or eating the wrong foods for your metabolism. It's often a food you just can't let go of (a little cream in the coffee, perhaps?), but really need to. I urge you to follow my plan. It is guaranteed to work every time. Don't stop following these principals until you have lost all that fat you have been hating for years. Your weight gain (or lack of weight loss) is not all your fault. Serving sizes (food choices, too) are mostly to blame, and I'm going to show you why.

PORTIONS VS. SERVINGS

According to the Cornell University Food and Brand Lab (a great site full of very interesting information that I urge you to go to: foodpsychology.cornell.edu):

- Serving sizes have grown four times larger since 1950.
- Dinner plate size has grown 36 percent between 1960 and 2007.
- A Serving of food served at home is now 33 percent larger than it was in 1996.
- Portion sizes can be 2 to 8 times larger than USDA or FDA serving-size suggestions.
- The average woman has increased her weight by 24.5 pounds since 1950.
- The average man has increased his weight by 28.5 pounds since 1960.
- Chocolate chip cookies have quadrupled in size.
- The average pizza slice grew 70 percent in calories between 1982 and 2002
- Caesar salads have doubled in calories.

The problem starts with who decides what and how much you should be eating. We are in trouble as a nation and in the middle of one of the biggest obesity epidemics that has reached crisis levels because the wrong people are deciding and telling us what a serving size should be. And guess who is making these decisions? WE are. That's right; the serving size typically seen on nutrition labels (1 slice of bread, 15 chips, 1 tablespoon of oil, an ounce or 1/4 cup of almonds, four cookies, 100 grams, half a bottle, etc.) is determined by how much the *typical* American over the age of four consumes in a single seating. Such questions were asked via national surveys, the Nationwide Health and Nutrition Examination Surveys, in the

1970s and 1980s by the USDA Center for Nutrition Policy and Promotion and then averaged out and determined by federal researchers. (In 2005 this same group began trying to update

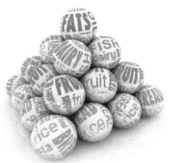

those sizes, but they are far from finished as we go to press.) That number was then rubberstamped on packages to make comparison shopping easier. It's not based on what you *should* eat and it's not meant to be a portion-size suggestion. It's more of a simple gauge to aim for, with the assumption that you'll eat less if you're trying to lose weight.

I don't know about you, but even when I was little I ate more than the average American (I don't and never did have a shut off valve or a body that intuitively knows when to stop). Or what about your obese neighbor who eats more for

---

WHAT TO KNOW ABOUT LABELS AND SERVING SIZE

To keep your metabolism running at optimal speeds and keep the weight off, remember this:

- **The serving sizes you see on a Nutrition Facts Panel are based on servings commonly eaten and they are not necessarily a recommendation. The serving sizes on a label are standardized so that you should be able to compare one product to another—a slice of bread from one brand to another. They are nothing more than a tool with which to compare different brands and versions of the same product.**
- **Always look at the label so that you know how many calories and other nutrients are in the package that you purchased, but don't use it as a guide for how much to eat. Eat at most half of what you think you should or don't eat it at all.**
- **Assume that all packages are more than 1 serving.**
- **When in doubt, don't eat it. If you have to ask yourself, you already know the answer.**

---

breakfast than she is supposed to eat in whole day? All of a sudden a serving size can be skewed to something quite large. This isn't a good way or a scientific way to determine what these numbers should be for a tool that you would think is to help keep us healthy and keep our weight within a healthy range. It's easy to see how we got into trouble in the first place, but it's only the beginning of the problem.

The first thing you can do is not assume the suggested serving size is the portion size. Serving size was created for manufacturers to create (hopefully) accurate and uniform nutrition labels across brands for comparison shopping. Use serving size as a rough gauge. Eat 1/2 or less of what's suggested. Can't stop eating once you start? Don't eat that particular food at all.

Even the director of the USDA Center for Nutrition Policy and Promotion, Dr. Robert Post, agrees. He has been quoted in several interviews available online stating; "You've got servings related to the nutrition facts panel and then another issue is a reasonable portion of food to build a healthy eating pattern. That may be a little different. The serving size might be bigger than what we'd use in the nutrition world to promote good habits."

> **IF YOU CAN'T PORTION CONTROL A CERTAIN FOOD DON'T EAT IT!**

May be a little different? *Might be bigger*? How are you supposed to know this? When I turn around and try to teach people real portion size I often get looks of disbelief, if not outright laughs of incredulity. Seriously. I feel the same way. It's kind of a betrayal. You think you're eating right, reading labels, but you're still stuck and not losing weight.

The system needs to be fixed. Meanwhile, how do you make informed choices regarding your health and weight loss? The deeper issue that needs to be faced is that portions are out of control, and a serving size is often bigger than a portion. Serving size, portion. How are you supposed to know how much to eat? You need to adjust your portions, especially if you have more than 10 pounds to lose. You need to accept these metabolism boosting laws as your weight-loss gospel. The worst thing that can happen to you when following this system is that you lose too much weight too fast. Wouldn't that be awful?

Fast weight loss isn't unhealthy when you follow *The Metabolism Solution*. My program is full of health-generating nutrition compared to incorrect and unbalanced diets that

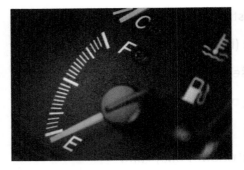

lack protein or deny all carbohydrates. The only carbs you should be afraid of are the ones that have labels on them. Vegetables are the only food that we under-eat on.

When it comes to figuring out how much you should be eating, think of yourself like a car's gas tank. It the tank only holds 10 gallons, then you can only put 10 gallons in. Period. It doesn't matter how slow or fast your metabolism is. The limit is the limit. Doesn't matter how high-end the gasoline is either (or how healthy the food is), you cannot add more. You can only add more gasoline when you burn up some of the gas already in your tank.

So how do you figure out a label and know portion size? For the fastest and easiest road to weight loss follow the serving and portion sizes in this book. Nevertheless, weigh and measure everything that goes into your mouth. Make a game out of it, it's not a punishment.

Many of these portion sizes are going to seem small if not downright tiny. I'm not particularly fond of them either. But I also know that in order to lose weight you need to abide by God's laws and learn to eat to fill your body's gas tank. Be honest and stop making excuses. Even "I only ate a little!" can sabotage you. Excuses are like telling your 10-gallon gas tank why it's okay that you're trying to squeeze in 15 gallons. You know what happens—the excess gas pours out all over the car no matter how expensive the gas is. Unfortunately the excess food we eat doesn't just dribble away off our bodies.

Knowing your numbers (food portions and calories, e.g.) is the way to boost your metabolism and lose weight for good. But better yet is eating food that doesn't come with labels. Avoid the foods where you find these labels and you won't have to determine what a reasonable portion size is for yourself. Eat fresh foods from the earth as much as you can. And if you are reading labels, always go for less—half—than the serving size suggestion states. Once you have reached your goals following *The Metabolism Solution* to a T, then—and only then—cautiously and slowly you can try adding back some of the foods you love. Just never stop drinking a protein shake for breakfast.

You almost need a Ph.D. in label science or a nutritionist on speed dial to really comprehend what or how much you're supposed to eat. To keep the weight off, keep it simple and stick to fish and lots of veggies.

WHAT HAS REPLACED THE FOOD PYRAMID?

If you're carrying extra weight around, scoring high on the BMI chart, and your scale is telling you to lose a few or more than a few, than your portion sizes are too big. Portions have become supersized over the years and most people no longer know how much food they are actually shoveling into their mouths. Knowing the proper 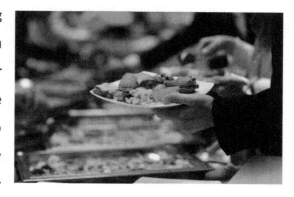 portion size can help stop you from packing on extra calories as well as extra pounds.

The decision of when and what to eat should be based on what your body needs, not what you feel like. The quantity of food you choose should always be based on your age, gender (males and growing children may need more than females), your level of physical activity, body mass index, and what you're about to do. For example, if you're going to bed you really can skip the food as your body is going to sleep and doesn't need many calories to do so. Now if you are going to the gym or about to move furniture around, your body may need *some* extra calories. In fact, you'll end up burning excess fat as fuel instead of your last

PORTIONS, SERVINGS, AND THE METABOLISM SOLUTION

How do I know how many "servings" of vegetables and fruit are right for me?
You want to find *your* right balance. For instance, if you are 5 feet tall and slight of frame, you will likely need fewer total servings of food than someone that might be over 6 feet tall and very active all day. There are plenty of professional recommendations out there as to what you "should" eat. Consider that this is not about finding the right rules, but rather choosing foundational principles to live by for your own optimal health. You know what works by what the scale shows. Keeping track of your body weight and journaling exactly what and how much you eat is critical so you can see cause and effect on the scale and know which foods you need to cut.

Why do you recommend so many servings of vegetables?
In the world of nutritional science, scientists might disagree about which foods are best to consume, but all agree that vegetables (organic preferably) are good for you. These recommendations are based on the fact that vegetables (especially green leafy ones) are the best way to lose belly fat. Vegetables are delicious nutritional powerhouses that stimulate the fat-burning process and keep you healthy.

If white fish is so healthy, why can't I eat as much as I want?
Your body can only digest a certain amount of protein from each meal (a rough gauge puts it at approximately 24 to 30 grams). Any excess you eat—no matter how healthy—is stored as fat to be used later. This occurs when overeating on any type of protein, even a lean, clean protein like white fish.

Remember the gas tank analogy? If your 5 feet tall your gas tank is totally different from the one your 6 foot tall husband has. If you eat the same amount, even though your husband's gas tank is larger, you gain weight no matter how fast your metabolism is. It's very simple; eat only what you need and you lose weight every time. Not losing? You're eating. I know it's brutal, but it's honest and the sooner you accept this the faster you'll lose weight. Don't beat yourself up when you overeat, just jump back on the plan or drink more shakes the next day instead of fussing over what to eat—when or how much—and dealing with the portion struggle.

What's the best way to find my portion size?
How do you know if your portions are too big? You weigh them using a food scale. Don't guess and don't trust your eye. Weigh the food you eat.

meal if you don't over feed your body. Keep in mind that if you are 20 pounds or more overweight, you won't starve if you don't eat a lot before a workout or higher activity levels. If your total body fat measures at 10 percent or under, you need to add calories before a workout to keep your body from chewing up muscle. But if you're over 10 percent body fat (and most of us are), you don't need to worry.

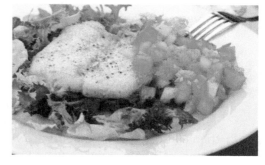

In 2011, the U.S. Department of Agriculture replaced the older food pyramid (we were actually less overweight when the food pyramid was invented) with a new symbol that dictates the recommended servings for each food group. The new food guide is called "The Dinner Plate." As its name would indicate, this is a dish-shaped icon, divided into five sections and labeled with the essential food groups: fruits, vegetables, grains, proteins, and dairy. This breakdown of types of food to eat may be fine for those maintaining, but in trying to lose weight it doesn't work.

So why replace the pyramid in the first place? Most nutritionists maintain (and I agree) that the pyramid was a misrepresentation of healthy eating, as it failed to differentiate nutrient-dense foods, like whole grains and fish, from empty-calorie foods such as refined cereals and pasta. All foods are not good for all people. How do you know if foods affect you differently or slow your metabolism? You know. Try this little self-test: What are the five foods that come to mind right now? Most likely it's the ones you wonder if you'll be able to eat—and these are most likely the ones you should avoid. Abstaining is easier than fighting with food you can't portion control. Try it, you'll see.

The one thing I agree on with the USDA is that vegetables should take up the majority of your plate. I say even more than the new plate depicts. The new guidelines also stress adding more "color" to your dish, and there is no better way to do this than eating your veggies. Color and texture are critical because we eat with all of our senses and vegetables provide both.

THESE WORDS MAY NOT MEAN WHAT YOU THINK THEY MEAN

IF IT SAYS WHOLE GRAIN—REFRAIN. All grains start their lives as whole grains, complete with a fully intact seed that includes three separate components. However, refining grains tends to remove the two outermost parts of the seed, stripping much of the grain's protein and at least 17 key nutrients. Whole grains have some protein, fiber, and many important vitamins and minerals that refined grains often lack. "Whole Grain" on a label means that it must have the same amount of all three seed components as a freshly harvested kernel. Words like "bran," "wheat germ," and "fiber" do not mean a product is whole grain. Check the ingredients: If the first ingredient contains the word "whole," then it's likely (though not guaranteed) that the product is mostly whole grain. If only the second ingredient contains the word "whole," then the product may contain anywhere from 1 percent to 49 percent whole grain. With multigrain breads, it can be even harder to know how much of it is truly whole grain. If you want to be completely confident that you're eating whole grains, look for a Whole Grain Stamp. If a product has a 100% Stamp, then all the grain ingredients are whole grains and it contains at least a full serving (16 grams) of whole grains. A Basic Stamp means the product has at least 8 grams (a half serving) of whole grains, though it may also have refined grains.

CHOLESTEROL-FREE DOESN'T MEAN GOOD FOR YOU OR GOOD FOR WEIGHT LOSS. Cholesterol is naturally found in foods like red meat (yes even lean chicken has some), dairy, egg yolks, and fish (shellfish mostly, not white fish). Research now suggests that eating foods that naturally contain cholesterol may not contribute to high blood cholesterol levels as much as was once thought. Many foods that are labeled cholesterol-free never would have contained cholesterol to begin with – but labeling them this way can trick you into thinking you're buying something healthy. It's more important to look at *fat* and *calories*—and *especially sugars*.

ZERO TRANS FATS DOES NOT MEAN YOU WON'T GAIN FAT. Trans fats are a dangerous type of fat often used in baked goods, frozen foods, frostings, coffee creamers, and microwavable popcorns, among many other foods. They are a major contributor to weight gain and heart disease and have already been banned or eliminated from many foods and restaurants. But beware: Current labeling guidelines allow Zero Trans manufacturers to say that any food that contains less than 0.5 grams of trans fats per serving contains "Zero Trans Fats." Even small amounts of these fats (like the amount you splash into your coffee everyday) can add up over time to severely damage your blood vessels and heart— not to mention make you gain weight because they slow down your metabolism. To make sure you're avoiding trans fats entirely, watch out for foods that list partially hydrogenated oil, hydrogenated vegetable oil, and shortening on their ingredients list. These foods contain trans fats.

LIGHTLY SALTED DOESN'T MEAN IT WON'T MAKE YOU RETAIN WATER OR GAIN WATER WEIGHT. If a food says it is "lightly salted," that generally means that it has 50 percent less sodium than the amount in a similar reference food, which does not necessarily make it low in sodium. To keep track of how much salt you're actually eating, check out the amount of sodium on the label and try to stay under 2,300 mg a day. People with certain health conditions may need to stick to low-sodium foods, which contain no more than 140 mg of sodium per serving. Retaining water is the reason the scale can go up so fast. Eat more asparagus and drink more water to offset that water retention, and you'll be fine by day's end. A good sweaty workout doesn't hurt, either.

"NOW WITH LESS FAT"—AND YOU'LL STILL GAIN WEIGHT. Foods that advertise as being "reduced fat" contain at least 25 percent less fat than a similar reference food does. However, less fat can mean less flavor and less satisfaction, and you might wind up eating more because you think you can. Manufacturers often try to make up for this lack of flavor-satisfaction by adding sugar and sodium. You may be tempted to eat more of the reduced-fat food, leaving you with a bigger waistline than if you stuck with the original and ate a little less.

SELL-BY DATES. Terms like "sell by," "use by," and "best before" are usually not good indicators of how safe the food is to eat. Rather than referring to when the food is safe to eat, these terms are simply suggestions from the manufacturer for when the food is at its peak quality. The "sell by" date tells grocery stores how long to offer the product for sale, and food is usually fresh for at least several days after that date. "Best by" usually speaks to when the food has its best flavor and quality. "Use by" is the last date recommended for use of the product at its peak quality. Confusion over these dates prompts 9 out of 10 Americans to throw away food before they really need to—a waste of taste and money. Freezing foods changes all of this. Freeze your Lean Bars and they last forever. Just remember to thaw them out before trying to bite into one.

DECODING THE FOOD LABEL

Let's get back to labels. Remember that just because you paid a lot for a food or it says that it "100% All Natural" and good for you does not mean it is good for weight loss. These so called health halo food such as "Whole grain" and "reduced fat" foods may not be what you think and are most often the reason we struggle with our weight. Marketers want us to believe we need to eat these foods, when in fact we don't.

Did you know that food labels often advertise healthy promises on the outside that the food on the inside may not keep? Learn which labels require a closer look with this easy-to-understand guide. I'm not actually suggesting that you eat these foods but I want you to know what they mean should you decide to indulge or justify on your food journal that what you ate was healthy. And don't assume these food shouldn't affect your weight loss. This couldn't be further from the truth.

There are so many misconceptions out there when it comes to food and weight loss. Cheese, peanut butter, nuts, and yogurt being good sources of protein is one that comes to mind. Or maybe you were one of the unlucky ones that saw on TV how avocados could help

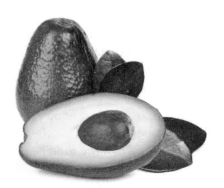 you shrink your thighs because they contain a "good" fat? While these foods may contain some nutrients like protein or fats, they aren't the best sources of protein and the fats aren't essential; therefore, these foods aren't the best for weight loss. You usually need to over eat on them to get the nutrients you need, and unless you are extremely physically active (even I don't qualify for this level), you'd be getting more calories than you need so they would cause weight gain or at the very least stop your weight loss.

You know slacking on exercise, not drinking enough water, or not getting enough

sleep slows weight loss. But a big culprit is falling off the eating plan, be it a weekend, one day, or for a meal. When cheating, you might eat too much of a food you shouldn't, or even following *The Metabolism Solution* you may not pay meticulous attention to what and how much you are supposed to eat. Then there's one of the most serious threats to weight loss; eating out.

When we eat out we tend to slip up on rich dressings and toppings like grated cheese, bacon bits, and croutons. You burn 300 calories by walking for three miles, but when you eat a 300-calorie muffin when you meet a friend for coffee, you totally erase the effect of your workout. *The Metabolism Solution* is a healthy, calorie-controlled meal plan that's complete with exercise to help maximize calorie burning and encourage permanent weight control. But if you blow off the rules, even one meal off the plan, you can trash a whole week's worth of effort. Don't think you can be lax with your calories because you exercise, and don't resist becoming lax about exercise just because you're cutting calories. Keep the following in mind the next time you say; "I only ate a little!" It's still too much.

Want to know what else may be stopping your weight loss? Eating foods that are higher in carbs, sugars, and fats than you think they are. Below are my rules for decoding labels.

The Food Label Reading Rules

Rule #1. If it's not on *The Metabolism Solution* food list it is not good for weight loss even though it may be good for you.

Rule #2. Don't pay any attention to those marketing claims on the front of the food packages. What the back label says counts most. The front of a label is created to sell not educate. The back is where the truth lies.

Rule #3. The highest number listed on the back label is what determines what nutrient category that food falls under because it contains the most of that nutrient. So if a food is a source of protein, protein should be the highest number you see listed on the label.

Guess which food I'm talking about here. According to its label it is a health food, yet it stops you from losing weight—not because it's bad for you, but because it's one of those "jack of all trades master of none" foods. Is it a protein? A carbohydrate? Something else? Millions of dieters enjoy it every day for breakfast or lunch and still don't see their waistlines shrinking. Are you wondering what that food is? Its yogurt. Don't get me wrong, yogurt has a place in our lives; I eat it just about every day, but as a *healthy dessert*. Why a dessert? It doesn't have enough protein to qualify for a metabolic-boosting meal and has too much sugar. As a dessert it delivers some nutrition and satisfies me.

> 4 GRAMS OF SUGAR = 1 TSP OF SUGAR. SO WHEN A FOOD ITEM CONTAINS 16 GRAMS OF SUGAR, YOU'RE EATING 4 TEASPOONS OF SUGAR. KEEP IN MIND THAT MOST MEAL-REPLACEMENT PROTEIN BARS AND PROTEIN SHAKES HAVE *AT LEAST* THAT MUCH. CHECK EVERY LABEL ON THE FOODS YOU EAT FOR SUGAR AS SUGAR STOPS WEIGHT LOSS. YOU WILL FIND IT IN THE MOST UNSUSPECTING PLACES—AND IN LARGE AMOUNTS.

Always check your labels to make sure you are eating the most metabolic-boosting foods. Don't forget to ask yourself; does this food serve a nutritional purpose? Everything we eat either boosts our metabolism or slows it down—choose wisely.

	Nonfat Greek Yogurt	Protein Bar	Sports Drink	LynFit Lean Bar
Serving Size	150 g	50 g	500 ml	50 g
Calories	100	180	120	150
Fat Calories	0	40	0	30
Total Fat	0	4.5 g	0	2.5 g
Saturated Fat	0	3 g	0	2 g
Protein	12g	20 g	0	19 g
Cholesterol	10 mg	15 mg	0	2.2 mg
Total Carbs	14 g	17 g	29 g	21 g
Fiber	< 1 g	2 g	0	10 g
Net Carbs	13 g	15 g	29 g	11 g
Sugar	13 g	2 g	29 g	2.5 g

ASK YOURSELF BEFORE YOU REACH FOR IT

1. How many servings are in the container and can you stop at 1 portion?

2. How many grams of protein does it contain per serving and keep in mind a perfect serving of protein is between 20 and 24 grams. In order to be considered a protein it needs to have that much.

3. How much sugar does it contain per serving? Look for *all* sugars—including sugar from agave, honey, or any and all natural sources. All sugars count. Aim for none or the lowest number you can find. Splenda and Truvia don't count because they won't affect your insulin levels.

4. How many carbohydrates does it contain per serving? Aim for the lowest carbs possible: less than 20 grams per serving unless it's a leafy green vegetable. If it is above 20 grams, it is a carb and should be limited.

5. How much fat does it contain per serving? Aim for the lowest number possible and don't eat the food if it contains more than 5 grams of fat per serving—unless its salmon.

   Of course calories count. Check to see how many calories the food item contains and do the math for each serving, counting calories and grams, to make sure you do not go over your daily requirement.

   IF you follow the above rules it brings the calories down for you.

TOP TEN FOOD SINS YOU CAN AVOID IF YOU READ THE LABELS

Now we're down to the nitty-gritty. The foods listed here, even if you only have a little bit of

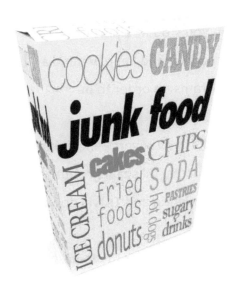

them, will affect your metabolism. It's not just about calories but the metabolic affect that these foods have on our waistlines because they trigger an insulin response that stops weight loss every time. And many of these foods tend to trigger the same part of our brain as drugs (the addiction center), so we become addicted and usually eat too much. Even though you exercise and make sure there is enough room in your plan for it calorically, these foods will sabotage your weight loss.

Unfortunately, you can't count on your smartphone app to run all your numbers for you because they can be significantly off. The bottom line is that you won't get lean if you take the caloric numbers from these apps as your gospel. It is the quality of your calories that counts. Remember; better is better? You want to take in calories that will boost your metabolism, not just fill you up. This is oh-so especially important when you're trying to lose belly fat. Empty calories (processed foods are mostly empty calories) have no job to do, thus, they store as fat very easily compared to the clean food plan of The Metabolism Solution. Wanna know where empty calories go? Straight to your hips, thighs, and belly. Try eliminating these foods and watch what happens. I dare you!

> ASK YOURSELF: "DO I HAVE ROOM CALORICALLY FOR THIS FOOD?" YOU WANT TO TAKE IN CALORIES THAT **BOOST** YOUR METABOLISM, NOT JUST FILL YOU UP.

Food Sin #1: Feta Cheese, the "Low-Fat" Cheese

One tiny little cube (about the size of a die) contains 6 grams of fat. Who eats just 1 cube? With 15 grams of fat per day on *The Metabolism Solution*, you better not be adding any other fats to your meals if you reach for the cheese. I love cheese, but it is best used for weight-gain diets. That's the only time I suggest it. If you're serious about losing weight, skip the cheese.

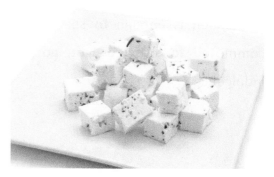

Food Sin #2: Oils

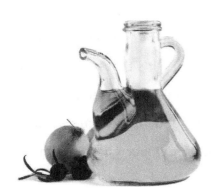

The 15 grams of fat a day rule is very important when it comes to losing weight and fat especially. One tablespoon of oil has 120 calories and 14 grams of fat. Doesn't leave much fat to have the rest of the day, does it? Even if you use a little, it's probably still too much. Use sprays or learn how to use chicken broth in cooking and stick to vinegar on your salads. Salad dressings will undo all the work you do by eating those healthy vegetables. You can't lose body fat if you keep eating lots of fats, even the "good ones". You'll continuously be replenishing your fat supply before you can burn what you already have.

Food Sin #3: Ice Cream

The serving size for ice cream is 1/2 cup. Who eats only that much? Who can't go through a pint of ice cream in one sitting? That one recommended serving will set you back

250 calories, 13 grams of fat, and 30 carbohydrates, all of which come from sugar. Even one tablespoon is enough to set you back. If you absolutely have to indulge and you are committed to losing weight, go for low-fat, sugar-free frozen yogurt. That is my true indulgence.

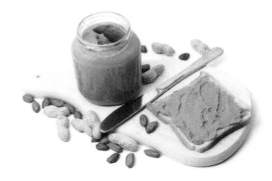

Food Sin #4: Peanut Butter

Peanut butter is a dieter's worst enemy because it is so deceptive. Most women eat one tablespoon of it straight out of the jar. In two tablespoons (the serving recommendation), you get 17 grams of fat and only 8 grams of protein.

More grams of fat than protein. Guess what? It's a fat and stop calling it anything else. Stop licking that peanut butter spoon and you can lose 8 pounds in a year—it's that big of a deal. Quit eating peanut butter all together and lose even more weight. Peanut butter is best for underweight hikers who need to eat a lot of calories. It's not good for the metabolism because it is not a complete protein and contains too much fat. Remember our 15-grams-a-day-of-fat rule?

Food Sin #5: Coffee Creamer, aka that Dash of Milk

This was the hardest thing for me to give up. No matter how little you use or how "insignificant" you may feel the amount is, it can hold you back from your weight loss goals. Do a test and see for yourself. The scale will tell all. It's not about the calories but where they come from, and look at what this stuff is

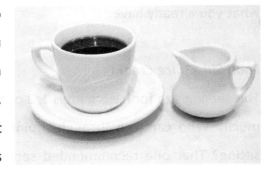

made of. All the fat and sugar in creamers can't make muscle or nourish eyes or skin or hair. There isn't one nutritious ingredient in here. Your body is left wondering, "What do you want me to do with this stuff?" So guess where it goes? Straight to your hips, thighs, and belly. Giving it up is worth it when you see how much better you look and feel and how much time you save in the gym.

Food Sin #6: Bread and Pasta

These two tie for 6th pace. Bread and pasta are nothing more than empty carbs that will need to be burned off in the gym. If you're serious about losing weight, stay away from these high-carb, high-calorie foods. Even at their recommended serving size they are over the limit in carbs and

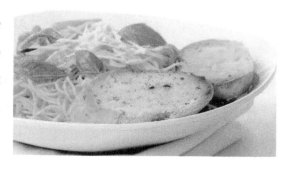

calories. Can you stick to one portion? One slice of bread? (hope you like open-faced sandwiches) or 1/2 cup of cooked pasta? (Remember, the portion is often smaller than the recommended serving size). In a 2-ounce serving as recommended by some pasta labels (Who even knows how much that is? Do you?), you get at least 200 calories and 35 to 40 carbohydrates per serving. Some pastas even have fat. It would take you one hour to burn that off in the gym—and that's if you only ate one portion. Bread is a metabolic nightmare. It doesn't matter how healthy or artisanal it is, or how much you paid for it. Limit it and you'll lose faster; it truly is that

100% NATURAL * 17g PROTEIN PER SLICE

NUTRITION FACTS	Amount /Serving	% Daily Value*	Amount/Serving	% Daily Value*	
	Total Fat 7g	11%	Total Carbohydrate 24g	8%	*Percent Daily Values are based on a 2,000 calorie diet. your daily values may be higher or lower depending on your calorie needs.
	Trans Fat 0g		Dietary Fiber 4g	16%	
Serving Size 1 Slice (65g)	Saturated Fat 1g	5%	Sugar 7g		Calories 2,000 2,500
Serving Per Container 13	Cholesterol 0mg	0%	Protein 17g		Total Fat Less than 65g 80g
	Sodium 360mg	15%			Sat Fat Less than 20g 25g Cholesterol Less than 300mg 300mg Sodium Less than 2,400mg 2,400mg Total Carbohydrate 300g 300g
Calories 230 Calories from Fat 60	Vitamin A 0% * Vitamin C 0%	*	Calcium 10% * Iron 10%		Dietary Fiber 25g 30g Calories per gram: Fat 9 * Carbohydrate 4 * Protein 4

INGREDIENTS: GRAIN MIXTURE (SPRING WHEAT, WINTER WHEAT, SOFT WHITE WHEAT, CORN GRITS, BARLEY GRITS, STEEL CUT OATS, CRACKED RYE, MILLET, FLAX SEEDS, SESAME SEEDS, SUNFLOWER SEEDS), WATER, WHEY PROTEIN ISOLATE, VITAL GLUTEN, WHOLE WHEAT FLOUR, MOLASSES, HONEY, RYE FLOUR, BROWN SUGAR, CANOLA OIL, SALT, CONTAINS 2% OR LESS OF YEAST. **CONTAINS: WHEAT AND MILK. MANUFACTURED IN A FACILITY THAT USES NUTS AND SOY.**

simple. Bread can set you back 170 calories per slice (and some breads recommend 2 slices per serving) and 21 carbs. No matter how much protein a bread label may claim, it will always have more carbs. Bread can never be a protein. It is a carb. See the label above? Look at all the sugar. Notice that the carb number is significantly larger than the protein number? Breads are almost always diet deceivers. Giving up bread will move that dial on the scale. I guarantee it.

Food Sin #8: Yogurt

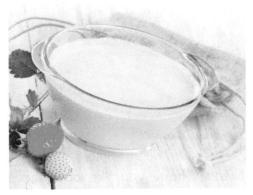

Ah, yogurt. I love the stuff. Yogurt, like most dairy, is an incomplete protein, loaded with sugar, fats, and all kinds of unknowns that slow your metabolism. I've managed to keep it in my diet by treating it as a dessert. I can't tell you how many stories I hear from people telling me how they struggle in trying to lose weight. Guess what they're eating for breakfast? Some so-called sugar-free, healthy yogurt. Yes, nonfat, sugar-free yogurt is better than ice cream, but it is never going to be a complete protein and will never beat the Complete Protein Shake for title of Metabolic-Boosting Breakfast.

I have a kid's size yogurt just about every day as dessert from my local frozen yogurt place. It keeps me feeling full and

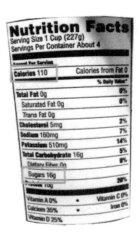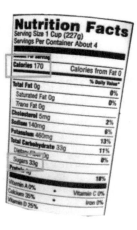

satisfied and I don't feel like I'm on a diet. In fact, ever since I started this habit I have never been more on track with my eating in my life. I feel alive and part of the world—and I don't miss ice cream anymore. In this day and age there are all kinds of frozen yogurt stands no matter where you are. Aim for the smallest size available, and if it's self-serve, simply count 1 Mississippi, 2 Mississippi, 3 Mississippi and you should get three ounces which is a portion. Always look for the lowest calories and sugar, and make sure it's nonfat so it is cleanest and won't slow your metabolism.

Take a look at the labels above. This small serving of a so-called healthy high-protein yogurt has 33 grams of carbohydrates, and it's all from sugar—that's 8 and 1/4 teaspoons of sugar. The label also specifies 0 grams of fat, but the ingredients list states it is made from whole milk solid, which definitely has fat.

Food Sin #9: Pizza

I have never met anyone who can eat just 1 slice of pizza. Every Monday morning I hear at least one of my clients complaining about lack of weight loss only to admit it was pizza night

on Friday. Pizza is better for weight gaining and never works for weight loss. You favorite pie is one of the highest calorie foods per ounce, full of fats and carbs. Don't buy into the claim that you're getting all your food groups or that it's loaded with vegetables and so is healthy. Avoid Pizza. The

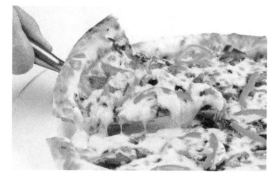

vegetables on it may be healthy on their own, if they're not prepared in fat, but not when smothered in cheese and placed on bread. The meats usually found on pizza are far too high in fat as well to count as sufficient protein to offset the carbs and fats already in the pizza. How many times have you blotted your pepperoni pizza slice before eating it? Think that's good for weight loss?

I can hear you from here: What about moderation? If you're at goal and doing fine maintaining, then every now and then (and limiting yourself to two slices) might be okay. But if you are struggling, pizza isn't going to help matters. Two plain cheese slices will set you back 740 calories, 36 grams of fat, and 72 grams of carbs—that's more than two days' worth of fat and carbs and three extra hours at the gym. Even one slice is too much. Yes, even thin crust pizza. Did you know that thin crust is just as high in carbohydrates? It's just rolled thinner. Don't think of thin crust pizza as a low-calorie alternative. It's not.

Food Sin #10: Alcohol

They may grow the grapes in California, but I think Fairfield County in Connecticut is the wine-drinking capital of the United States. I run into so many people who defend their nightly glass

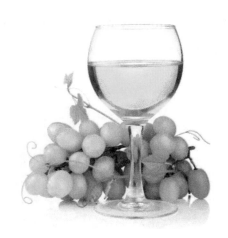

of Merlot and refuse to take it out of their diet—all while ranting about how they just can't lose those last pounds or that spare tire around their middles. Wine has nutritional value, they argue, containing minerals and antioxidants. But so do vegetables—and more of them. Wine is a big factor especially when it comes to belly fat. Why is that? Because alcohol has almost two times the amount of carbs as sugars. Wine is a carbohydrate full of empty calories. A glass of wine can contain from 9 to 19 grams of carbs per serving; flavored wines can have even more. And who follows the serving size when pouring a glass? Do you even know what it is?

In some cases a slightly sweet and low-alcohol wine may have fewer calories than a dry high-alcohol wine. But you'd be hard pressed to know for sure since wine doesn't come with labels. Neither do other kinds of alcohol. No calorie counts, no grams of carbohydrates—

not even serving suggestions. And guess why? Because wine and liquors are not considered part of a daily diet. They are not required to by law. Perhaps labels should be required? You can dig around to find calorie and "nutritional" information, but it would be much easier if it were on the bottle.

> WHEN IT COMES TO YOUR DAILY CALORIES, WOULD YOU RATHER EAT A SALAD LOADED WITH VEGETABLES THAT WILL FILL YOU UP OR HAVE A GLASS OF WINE THAT WILL LEAVE YOU HUNGRY?

When it comes to a glass of wine, which is a 6-ounce serving, calories can range anywhere from just over 100 (for a sweet white wine low in alcohol) to almost 300 (for a sweet dessert wine). Popular types like Merlot and Chardonnay tend to fall in the 150-to-200-calorie range per glass. When it comes to your daily calories, would you rather eat a salad loaded with vegetables that will fill you up or have a glass of wine that will leave you hungry?

Six

YOUR WORKOUT MAY BE SLOWING YOUR METABOLISM

These days, there are dozens—if not hundreds—of exercise programs for you to choose from. You can work out 24-hours a day at the never-closing gym, you can do cold yoga and hot yoga, train like a Navy S.E.A.L., stretch like a ballet dancer, twirl around a stripper's pole, and whatevericize away the fat. Where do you start? You know, you can lose weight—if you can control your food very specifically—*without* exercise. So why bother at all? I'll tell you why, to feel good. You want to tone up your arms for the dress you're wearing to your son's graduation. You want to be able to run after your toddler without getting out of breath. You want to sleep better. You want to find an outlet for the stress in your life. You want to move without your body aching. You want to reduce your risk of heart disease, high blood pressure, cancer, and diabetes. Need I go on?

Oh, and did I mention that exercise can turbo charge your metabolism? It's a sad fact that as you age, your metabolic rate (how quickly your body burns calories for fuel) slows down. Starting at about age 25, the average, not physically active person's metabolism declines between 5 and 10 percent per decade, which accumulates to a decline between 20 to 40 percent over an adult life span? However, there is good news for those who continue physical activity their whole lives: only a 0.3 percent metabolic decline per decade. Isn't that a good reason to keep moving? If your current fitness program isn't working, needs a jump start, keeps leaving you hurting, or if you don't have one at all, you've come to the right place.

Not all exercise is created equal, however. Metabolic Exercise is key to revving up your calorie-burning engine.   Simply put, metabolic training uses 8 to 10 specific multitasking moves (some use dumbbells) to work all the major muscle groups in every 30-minute workout no more than three times a week. You read it right: Not every day, but three days a week. Each move includes at least 2 large muscle groups per move and they always include a leg move so you triple your calorie burn in half the time. That's intensity. And there's no rest between moves, too. This is combined with daily aerobic walking I call the Metabolic Core Walk. You don't have to do all the moves in one session. You can break up a metabolic workout and do a little at a time throughout the day in your own home or even at an office. No gym membership required. No classes to run to. You just have to do it at your pace three times a week.

Almost sounds too good to be true, doesn't it? But it works.

YOU CANNOT EXERCISE AWAY A BAD DIET

TOO MUCH EXERCISE STRESSES YOUR BODY. TOO MUCH STRESS INCREASES YOUR CORTISOL LEVEL. TOO MUCH CORTISOL PUMPS UP THE SPARE TIRE AROUND YOUR MIDDLE.

Remember that when trying to lose weight, what you eat is at least 80 percent—no, scratch that, 90 percent if you're over 40—of your weight loss and exercise makes up the remaining 10 percent. You cannot eat whatever you want, whenever you want, or even have that "little" cheat splurge and expect an extra hour at the gym to make it all go away. Look at the numbers: To burn off that cheeseburger you'll need at least 6 more miles running on the treadmill or about 90 or more minutes walking. That so-called smoothie, which is really a milkshake in disguise, sets you back almost 900 calories—and it is really hard to burn 900 calories in one workout. There's lots of information out there on how many calories particular activities burn; it's rather sobering looking at the numbers.

Body Mass Index Table

BMI	19	20	21	22	23	24	25	26	27	28	29	30	31	32	33	34	35	36	37	38	39	40	41	42	43	44	45	46	47	48	49	50	51	52	53	54
	Normal						Overweight					Obese										Extreme Obesity														
Height (inches)												Body Weight (Pounds)																								
58	91	96	100	105	110	115	119	124	129	134	138	143	148	153	158	162	167	172	177	181	186	191	196	201	205	210	215	220	224	229	234	239	244	248	253	258
59	94	99	104	109	114	119	124	128	133	138	143	148	153	158	163	168	173	178	183	188	193	198	203	208	212	217	222	227	232	237	242	247	252	257	262	267
60	97	102	107	112	118	123	128	133	138	143	148	153	158	163	168	174	179	184	189	194	199	204	209	215	220	225	230	235	240	245	250	255	261	266	271	276
61	100	106	111	116	122	127	132	137	143	148	153	158	164	169	174	180	185	190	195	201	206	211	217	222	227	232	238	243	248	254	259	264	269	275	280	285
62	104	109	115	120	126	131	136	142	147	153	158	164	169	175	180	186	191	196	202	207	213	218	224	229	235	240	246	251	256	262	267	273	278	284	289	295
63	107	113	118	124	130	135	141	146	152	158	163	169	175	180	186	191	197	203	208	214	220	225	231	237	242	248	254	259	265	270	278	282	287	293	299	304
64	110	116	122	128	134	140	145	151	157	163	169	174	180	186	192	197	204	209	215	221	227	232	238	244	250	256	262	267	273	279	285	291	296	302	308	314
65	114	120	126	132	138	144	150	156	162	168	174	180	186	192	198	204	210	216	222	228	234	240	246	252	258	264	270	276	282	288	294	300	306	312	318	324
66	118	124	130	136	142	148	155	161	167	173	179	186	192	198	204	210	216	223	229	235	241	247	253	260	266	272	278	284	291	297	303	309	315	322	328	334
67	121	127	134	140	146	153	159	166	172	178	185	191	198	204	211	216	223	230	236	242	249	255	261	268	274	280	287	293	299	306	312	319	325	331	338	344
68	125	131	138	144	151	158	164	171	177	184	190	197	203	210	216	223	230	236	243	249	256	262	269	276	282	289	295	302	308	315	322	328	335	341	348	354
69	128	135	142	149	155	162	169	176	182	189	196	203	209	216	223	230	236	243	250	257	263	270	277	284	291	297	304	311	318	324	331	338	345	351	359	365
70	132	139	146	153	160	167	174	181	188	195	202	209	216	222	229	236	243	250	257	264	271	278	285	292	299	306	313	320	327	334	341	348	355	362	369	376
71	136	143	150	157	165	172	179	186	193	200	208	215	222	229	236	243	250	257	265	272	279	286	293	301	308	315	322	329	338	343	351	358	365	372	379	386
72	140	147	154	162	169	177	184	191	199	206	213	221	228	235	242	250	258	265	272	279	287	294	302	309	316	324	331	338	346	353	361	368	375	383	390	397
73	144	151	159	166	174	182	189	197	204	212	219	227	235	242	250	257	265	272	280	288	295	302	310	318	325	333	340	348	355	363	371	378	386	393	401	408
74	148	155	163	171	179	186	194	202	210	218	225	233	241	249	256	264	272	280	287	295	303	311	319	326	334	342	350	358	365	373	381	389	396	404	412	420
75	152	160	168	176	184	192	200	208	216	224	232	240	248	256	264	272	279	287	295	303	311	319	327	335	343	351	359	367	375	383	391	399	407	415	423	431
76	156	164	172	180	189	197	205	213	221	230	238	246	254	263	271	279	287	295	304	312	320	328	336	344	353	361	369	377	385	394	402	410	418	426	435	443

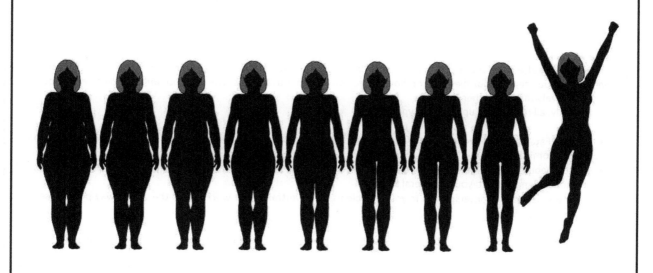

IT'S YOUR BMI THAT MATTERS
WHY BEING A LITTLE FAT IS GOOD—REALLY!

The bathroom scale is a standard tool for anyone trying to get into better shape, but the number it shows isn't the only one you need to pay attention to. You either dread or anticipate what that scale will say, but it's not the be-all and end-all when it comes to weight. It doesn't tell you the whole story. No one would argue it's a good idea to never step on a scale. It's important to keep tabs on your weight, but it's also important to understand what makes up your weight. That's where BMI comes in.

BMI stands for Body Mass Index, which refers to the amount of fat you have. The number is easy to figure out with a calculator: It's your weight in pounds divided by the square root of your height in inches and then multiplied by 703. (If you'd rather not do the math yourself, you can go to my website lynfit.com and use the online BMI calculator there.) Your fitness level is then assessed based on where this final number falls on the BMI chart, from underweight to extremely obese.

Your BMI paints a better picture of your health and fitness level than a scale alone. It tells you what you really need to know if you're serious about boosting your metabolism and changing the way you look and feel. For instance, you can reach your goal weight but find that with a high BMI you still don't look the way you want to in a bathing suit. Just because your lighter doesn't mean your leaner. If your BMI remains higher than it should be, your metabolism will be slow and you'll struggle to keep the weight off until you lower your BMI. And more importantly, if your BMI remains high, the greater the risk of developing obesity-related diseases, including heart disease, high blood pressure, stroke, and Type 2 diabetes.

Can you be *too* lean or fit and fat? Yes!

Being too lean is just as unhealthy as being overweight. If your BMI is too low, you are at greater risk for osteoporosis, infertility, malnutrition, thyroid problems and even hair loss. There is a certain amount of body fat, Essential Body Fat, which is necessary for you to stay healthy. Why? Essential Body Fat helps to regulate metabolism and body temperature, insulates organs, and helps with brain functioning, among other things. Fat, contrary to its bad reputation, is actually vital to our survival. It's involved in many important processes—even metabolizing carbohydrates.

Women need more fat than men—that's why they're curvier. The possibility of childbirth creates different hormonal demands on the female body which affects fat. Men have a different type of fat from women and store if differently.

For *basic* survival, women need 8% to 12% fat and men require 3% to 5%. Which end of the range you fall into as your optimum depends on your body structure and composition–i.e., are you small-, medium-, or large-framed? Your height, whether you build muscle easily, and whether you tend to keep lean muscle more than fat also determine which end of the range you fall into. It should come as no surprise that whether you eat right or work out shows up in your BMI.

Everything else over and above the essential body fat you have is storage fat. And how much excess fat you store depends on your genes, your diet, and on how active you are on a daily basis. *The Metabolism Solution* attacks stored fat more effectively than any other diet plan.

Basically, all fat is made up of three types of fat:

- Visceral Fat. It protects your internal organs but can be very bad for your health if you have too much packed in your abdominal cavity.
- Subcutaneous Fat. Generally the fat you can pinch and the one you must often want to get rid of. Unsightly as it is, it is not as dangerous to you as visceral fat.
- Intramuscular fat. It's interspersed in your muscle tissue. Overtraining or working out the wrong way predisposes you to this type.

Needless to say, you should not aim to get your overall body fat percentage any lower than your essential value—that would be dangerous. It is good to try and keep within your idea range.

Use the chart on the opposite page or a scale that tells you your BMI. Be consistent with the method you choose and track your BMI weekly. Your BMI will go down if you follow *The Metabolism Solution* as suggested.

I have hundreds, if not thousands, of client stories to pull from where someone tries to explain away why the scale isn't moving or perhaps has even gone in the wrong direction. There's a common theme with many of them: coming home from the gym starved and eating freely. You worked out hard and you've burned calories, so you deserve to eat. That's the reasoning. What it really is, however, is a case of over exercising.

> A LONG WORKOUT COULD LEAD TO A QUICK PIG-OUT.

It seems that lots of people out there are indeed trying to exercise away a bad diet. The media has coined it "Boomeritis" to explain the increase in Baby Boomers ending up in the emergency room from over-exercising. And it's not just Baby Boomers. You can't sit at your desk all week and then let a drill sergeant-like instructor yell at you and put you through paces meant for an 18-year-old boy. That's going to hurt. Now if these militaristic or other

THE ONE-MINUTE PUSHUP TEST

A pushup is the best way to determine your overall fitness—especially your upper body strength. Set a timer and go. Men use traditional pushup position, women can start on knees if needed. No clapping between pushups required. *(Developed by the American College of Sports Medicine, acsm.org)*

Women	Age 20-29	30-39	40-49	50-59	60-69
Excellent	30	27	24	21	17
Very Good	21-29	20-26	12-23	11-20	12-16
Good	15-20	13-19	11-14	7-10	5-11
Fair	10-14	8-12	5-10	2-6	2-4
Needs Improvement	9	7	4	1	1

Men	Age 20-29	30-39	40-49	50-59	60-69
Excellent	36	30	25	21	18
Very Good	29-35	22-29	17-24	13-20	11-17
Good	22-28	17-21	13-16	10-12	8-10
Fair	17-21	12-16	10-12	7-9	5-7
Needs Improvement	16	11	9	6	4

THE SLOW METABOLISM TEST

Do you have hard time losing weight? Do you feel flabby, fatigued, and fat? You may be struggling with a sluggish-slow metabolism and the good news is that no matter how much damage has been done from constant yo-yo dieting, eating the wrong foods, or lack of exercise, it can be fixed. How do you know if your metabolism is slow? Chances are that if you're reading this, you already know the answer to that question, but I suggest that you take The Metabolism Test to give you the answers you need to solve your weight-loss problems once and for all. It can be fixed and The Metabolism Solution *will show you how.*

Please answer with a simple yes or no.

- Do you have a hard time losing weight?
- Do you struggle with cravings for carbohydrate foods and sugar?
- Do you have to starve yourself in order to lose and ounce?
- Do you exercise but still can't lose weight?
- Do you carry excess pounds and fat specifically around your mid-section, hips and thighs?
- Do you have cellulite covering your body and on areas where cellulite typically does not go?
- Are you tired and sluggish most of the time?
- Are you female?
- Are you over 30?
- Have you been chronically stressed for more than 30 days?
- Do you drink more than 1 drink per week?
- Were your parents or grandparents overweight?
- Have you gone through peri-menopause or menopause?
- Are you considered short? (Under 5 feet 4 inches)?
- Is your waist size more than 35 inches (women) or 40 inches (men)?

- Do you have any of the following medical conditions that you are aware of?
  - High Blood Pressure (systolic over 130 or Diastolic over 85)?
  - High Cholesterol?
  - Low HDL (good) Cholesterol?
  - Allergies?
  - High Blood sugar (110 or higher)?
  - High Triglycerides (150 or higher)?
  - Depression/Anxiety?
  - Seizures?
  - Do you sleep less than 7 hours per night?
  - Have you been told that you have hypo or hyper thyroid by a Doctor?
  - Do you take medications to treat any of these ailments?
  - Do you retain water or feel bloated often?
  - Do you have at least one bowel movement every day?
  - Do you have food sensitivities? Gluten? Dairy? Fish?
- Have you gained more than 10 pounds in the last 2 years?
- Have you lost weight and regained it more than once in the last 2 years

- Do you think your metabolism is slow?

If you answered YES to 5 or more of these questions, your metabolism is slow and needs to be boosted in order for you to lose weight and feel great. The more YES's, the more critical it is. Even if you answered YES to fewer than 5 questions, it's still a good idea to add the suggestions outlined in these pages to keep your metabolism moving. The Metabolism Solution *is the answer to losing weight and preventing you from gaining weight as you age.*

methods are working for you, more power to you. But they didn't work for me and they aren't working for those I counsel every day.

The truth is over-exercising can make you think you want to eat or, perhaps more accurately, that you deserve to eat. Studies have shown that if you have a hard work out, you may than engage in some "compensatory eating," as it is called. And there goes all your hard work. **You only truly need one third of the calories you consume every day as it is.** Why add even more just because you're exercising? That's counterproductive.

> HOME WORKOUTS ARE MORE EFFECTIVE IN LESS TIME.

Over-exercising may not only give you a false sense of permission to eat, it may also stress you out. A long workout physically stresses your body—you're breathing hard, sweaty, maybe even have shaky limbs. And stress, regardless of the kind—good *and* bad stress—produces the same hormone: cortisol. As cortisol levels rise, your body has a propensity to store fat in your midsection and make it easier to gain weight.

Just last year Columbia University published a study, one of the largest of its kind on exercise and mental health, that found that if you exercise *less than* 2.5 hours a week you have a higher risk of depression, anxiety, injuries, and overall poor health. Conversely, the study found that exercising *more than* 7.5 hours a week can make you sick. You read that right. If you're going to the gym two hours a day or stressing over the fact that you can't squeeze it in, stop and keep reading.

> A METABOLIC WORKOUT NOT ONLY BLASTS FAT FASTER, BUT KEEPS BLASTING FAT FOR THE NEXT 36 HOURS.

METABOLIC EXERCISE VS. EVERYTHING ELSE

All exercise is better than no exercise, but Metabolic Exercise is better than others. You don't have to be a weekend warrior vomiting after a run (which is easier to do than you may think), a contortionist pulling muscles and then not being able to do *anything* for weeks while you heal, or a weightlifter trying to go toe-to-toe with the big boys at the gym and then finding yourself flat on your back with an ice pack and no comfortable position. You do not need to be super-sore to lose weight.

There is a better way. Metabolic exercise is the most effective way to force your body to burn calories at an accelerated pace, which helps you burn more fat while you exercise. If you google "metabolic exercise" you'll find many plans claiming to offer just that. Don't be fooled.

> THE BEST SECRET OF ALL: IF YOU EAT RIGHT YOU CAN EXERCISE LESS. The cleaner you eat the less you time you'll need to spend in the gym. You have to learn to eat for what you do. Sitting and watching TV? Guess what? You don't need food. Walking all day shopping? Don't listen to your head hunger, no big meals and definitely no binging required. You need protein, veggies, and carbs that will sustain your activity. Working out? Grab a Lean Bar or sip a Protein Shake as you go out the door. Or maybe nothing at all. If you eat on my plan you get exactly what your body needs, no more no less. And guess what happens when you eat what you need? You begin to burn fat no matter how slow your metabolism is.

If your current exercise takes more than 45 minutes a day to do, it's not metabolic. If you're growing your arms and legs when you're trying to lose inches and tone, it's not metabolic. If you're dancing for an hour—while it may be fun—it's not metabolic. No dumbbells? It's definitely not metabolic and it certainly won't strengthen your bones. You may not get the results you want using Pilates, yoga, or Zumba class, either. If you want to burn fat faster, buff up your arms, and slim down your legs, I have good news for you—especially if you are a busy person with barely 10 minutes to spare. A run may be a good idea (if your knees can take it), but a metabolic workout not only blasts fat faster, but keeps blasting fat for the next 36 hours. In 20 to 30 minutes of exercise you can rev up your metabolism for the next day and a half (a thermogenic diet helps). What makes my exercise different? It works every time, if you do it.

For your mental and physical health, you absolutely need to move every day. By now you've heard it a thousand times: take the stairs instead of the elevator, park just a little bit further away, walk during your lunch break, and so on. But you only need to do metabolic exercise three times a week—not more. The good news? One workout a week keeps you from backsliding; two workouts will get you results; but three will get you there the fastest. More than that, and it's overkill.

One of the things that stop a fitness plan dead in its tracks is lack of structure and lack of results. If you don't see results in two weeks, stop. When you are on the right track, you know right away if it's working: your clothes start to fit better, you don't ache, and you can do it and keep doing it for the rest of your life. If your routine is too hard are you going to be able to keep doing it? Are you going to want to? If it's too easy, how long are you going to spend your time with a plan that takes forever to show results?

Let's get back to dumbbells for a moment. If you're on a calorie-reducing diet that does not include strength training, then you are losing muscle. When you *increase* your muscle, as you do with strength training, you boost your resting metabolic rate—burning more calories even while resting. Lifting weights consumes calories, raises your metabolism, and builds muscles that consume extra calories later on so your body burns more calories even when doing nothing. A 2000 study by G.R. Hunter et al. found that subjects increased their resting metabolic rates after six months of resistance training and were burning an extra 100 calories a day. Cardio workouts also boost metabolism. In another study, this one by J.A.

THE PLANK TEST: CORE STRENGTH AND ENDURANCE

How strong is your core? A strong core keeps you free from injury and your back in tip-top shape for the rest of your life. If your core isn't strong enough, you're not fit enough. The Plank Test is not only a way to gauge your core's fitness. It's also what you need to do to get your core strong. Doing a plank two to three times a week (with one day between each), you can get fit fast.

Find an exercise mat or a comfortable spot on the floor and assume a pushup position but with your weight on your forearms instead of your hands. Contract your stomach muscles as if you're about to be punched. Now hold it. Your body should form a straight line from shoulders to ankles.

If you can't make it for one minute, you need to work on your core strength. The remedy is planks two to three times a week for as long as you can until you build up endurance. Over two minutes? You are strong.

Potteiger et al., participants who did moderate intensity cardio exercise three to five days per week, 20 to 45 minutes a time, for 16 months. These subjects increased their resting metabolic rate by burning an extra 129 calories a day. Imagine how walking every day will affect your body. I love the idea of burning an extra 100 calories a day while doing nothing, don't you?

More isn't better, better is better applies to fitness and supplementing more than you know, and the reason no one talks about it is that they usually want to sell you something. Whether it's a gym membership, expensive bulky equipment, or a trainer who wants you to depend on her while charging you more than you'd care to pay. These may not keep you lean. The secret to *living* lean and not just getting lean is that whatever gets you fitter and causes you to lose weight is also what keeps those pounds off. Exercise needs to fit into your life, not become your life.

I live in the real world. I'm a wife and mother and work crazy hours every week, I need the fastest, most effective workout that benefits me in the least amount of time. I'm betting that's what you need, too. Who has three or six hours a day to spend in the gym? Not me. That's why your diet needs to support your results.

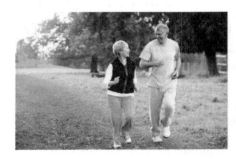

THE STARTING LINE

Most people have no clue where to begin when it comes to an exercise program. Starting is simpler than you think. Exercise is about more than weight loss; it's about making you stronger, more flexible, and cardio-vascularly fit. When you exercise, all kinds of miraculous things happen. Your immune system is stimulated; you're energized and detoxified; depression lifts; your skin gets tighter (especially if you're eating right); your bone density improves; and perhaps best of all aging is not only slowed but reversed. You can't make excuses when all this (and more) is on the line.

I always have new clients take a fitness test, one that I've developed over the years. Not only do I assess their physical ability, but I ask hard questions about their goals, activity, and mindset. You need to assess to know what you need to do and what you need to change to get there. I have my clients walk for 20 minutes, check their BMI score, do pushups and planks, and I check their flexibility. I ask them questions—like those in The Slow Metabolism Test—about their general health.

If all you are looking to do is just workout, there are so many options: P90X, insanity, Cross Fit, Zumba, and more. If you want more flexibility, then Pilates and yoga may be calling to you. But if you are looking to lose weight because your metabolism needs a kick start (and you'll know if you take The Slow Metabolism Test): it's time for a change. It's not you who has failed; your fitness program has failed you.

READY, SET, GO! THE 1-MILE WALK TEST

Get your walking shoes out. This test measures your aerobic (cardiovascular) fitness level based on how quickly you can walk one mile at moderate intensity. Warm up by walking slowly for a few minutes and when you are ready to begin, start the clock. At the end be sure to follow up with some stretches. Please don't try this unless you are regularly walking for 15 to 20 minutes several times a week. Times given in minutes and seconds. These standards are based on information from the American College of Sports Medicine (acsm.org).

Age	20-29	30-39	40-49	50-59	60-69	70+
Women						
Excellent	< 13:12	< 12:24	< 12:54	< 12:24	< 14:06	< 15:06
Good	11:54-13:00	12:24-13:30	12:54-14:00	13:24-14:24	14:06-15:12	15:06-15:48
Average	13:01-14:30	13:31-14:12	14:01-14:42	14:25-15:12	15:13-16:18	15:49-18:48
Fair	13:43-14:30	14:13-15:00	14:43-15:30	15:13-16:30	16:19-17:18	18:49-20:18
Poor	> 14:30	> 15:00	>15:30	> 16:30	> 17:18	>20:18
Men						
Excellent	< 13.12	< 13:42	< 14:12	< 14:42	< 15:06	< 18:18
Good	13:12-14:06	13:42-14:36	14:12-15:06	14:42-15:36	15:06-16:18	18:18-20:00
Average	14:07-15:06	14:37-15:36	15:07-16:06	15:37-17:00	16:19-17:30	20:01-21:48
Fair	15:07-16:30	15:37-17:-00	16:07-17:30	17:01-18:06	17:31-19:12	21:49-24:06
Poor	> 16.30	> 17:00	> 17.30	> 18.06	> 19.12	> 24.06

THE METABOLIC CORE WALK

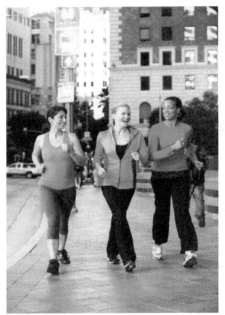

The first step, no pun intended, of a metabolic workout is the Metabolic Core Walk. Done daily, it strengthens your bones and heart and boosts your metabolism. The Metabolic Core Walk, a cardio workout, is the most important step in boosting your metabolism. If you did nothing but this walk for 45 to 60 minutes daily, you would change your body shape fast.

So what is it? Metabolic Core Walking is walking with good posture at a speed that revs up the calorie burn. That's not a casual stroll while window shopping and it's not a jog either. You should feel like you're gliding, not pounding the pavement. Walk forward gently as if you're pushing a carriage. The next time at you're at the market, get a feel for it when pushing your shopping cart down the aisles. It's walking with a sense of urgency, back straight, arms moving. Walk with your core—as if you're squeezing a golf ball in your buttocks and keeping your stomach muscles pulled in tight. Just don't confuse good posture with tensing your shoulders and raising them to your ears. Imagine God is pulling a string coming from your chest so you keep your neck nice and long and your shoulders back and down.

> **WHEN METABOLIC CORE WALKING, IMAGINE GOD IS PULLING A STRING FROM YOUR CHEST SO YOU KEEP YOUR NECK LONG AND YOUR SHOULDERS BACK AND DOWN.**

Start with 20 minutes a day until you can walk 5 miles in 60 minutes; you want to be able to walk a 15-minute mile without feeling like you're having a heart attack. And you don't have to do it all in one stretch. You can break it up, say, in 20-minute increments. That's it. Walking. Your knees will thank you and so will the rest of you. And you can walk anywhere, anytime. There's no need to ever step foot in a gym.

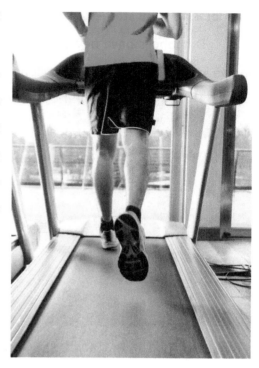

If it's pouring rain or snowing, I take it inside. Treadmills are great to keep you walking whatever the weather and even better at keeping you at a consistent speed. Those times when I'm having an off day (I get them, too), I jump on my stationary bike and ride longer (more than an hour) at a lower tension. (Many drafts of this book were read and edited while I pedaled away) The bike really helps if you can't walk due to injury but can still pedal. (It's crucial that you do not stop exercising in some capacity.) I'm not a fan of outdoor bikes for fat loss. Aside from weather factoring in whether you work out or not, you can't keep a consistent speed (because of the hills on the road and obstacles like cars and people) on an outdoor bike. Think of investing in a treadmill or stationary bike. With one, you can absolutely never use the excuse of "I couldn't walk today, it was too rainy."

DUMBBELLS FOR SMART WORKOUTS

Before you think it's inevitable that you'll end up with frail bones as you get older, consider that working out with weights in your hands at least twice a week strengthens your bones. Pilates, yoga, and dancing don't do that as effectively or efficiently. Twenty minutes a week can halt osteoporosis. Your bones need you to work out with weights. What are you waiting for? You don't need to spend $2,000 on some fancy machine with adjustable pulleys and cables. You don't need to join a gym. Dumbbells, hand weights—any brand that you can hold comfortably and purchase in

YOUR BONES NEED YOU TO WORK OUT WITH WEIGHTS!

your local discount store—will do. Even a can in a pinch.

Dumbbells have never gone out of fashion with those serious about fitness. The moves shown on the following pages will boost your metabolism. Looking at the pictures and reading

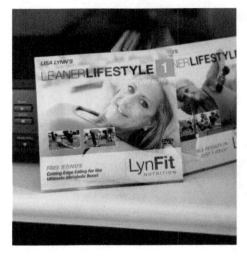

how-to descriptions can start you off, but you may want to get a copy of my LynFit DVDs (lynfit.com) as well so you can follow along and see exactly how they are done.

A metabolic workout may be quick compared to some workouts, but it is effective. It shouldn't kill you, but if it feels easy, you're not doing it right. Go deeper, squeeze harder and tighter. Add another set of reps or use heavier weights. Keep going. Each move combines three of your major muscle groups with minimal rest between. You will sweat, but you won't be left shaky and pale on the floor. Just because these exercises are good for your metabolism does not mean more exercise is better. Three times a week. Stick to the plan.

THE TOE TOUCH TEST

No other test is so easy or so telling. Can you touch your toes? If you can touch them, you will be about 300 percent *less* likely to lose your posture or have posture issues. Posture is everything when it comes to keeping your body healthy.

Do the test: Put your feet together, bend over, and reach for our toes. Your knees need to be kept straight. Can you touch your toes with straight knees? If you can, you pass; if not, you need to work on strengthening your core muscles and your flexibility. Follow the balanced workouts and stretches in this book to "correct" imbalances; other programs may actually cause muscle imbalances by overworking some muscles while not working others hard enough. A fit body is healthy body.

If you cannot reach your toes, you risk suffering from loss of spine posture—and the health of your body is determined by the health of your spine. That's why doctors have you bend over and touch your toes in a routine physical. With that one test, they can check your hamstrings, glues, abs, and hip mobility. A failed toe touch can lead to back problems and it lets you know you need the Recovery Stretch.

The 30-Minute Metabolic Workout

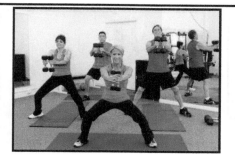

1. Deep Squat to Front Raise. Stand with feet shoulder width apart with dumbbells in hands in front. Squat down and stand back up raising dumbbells to chin level.

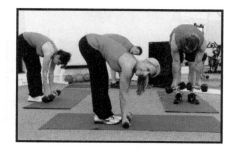

2. Stiff Leg Dead Lift. Stand with legs together, knees slightly bent, dumbbells in hands. Bend at waist lowering weights to the ground, using the back of the leg bring them back up to knee level.

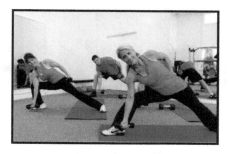

3. Side Lunge with Arm Curl. Lunge to side with weight in hand. Lower weight to lunging leg, pushing with your heel back to start position while simultaneously bringing dumbbell to your waist in a curl.

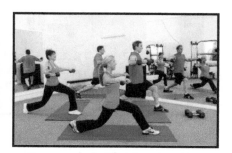

4. Front Lunge with Side Raise. Holding dumbbells in hand, step or lunge forward to front lunge position, perform side dumbbell raises or, in a front lunge position, perform side dumbbell raises (you decide which is best)

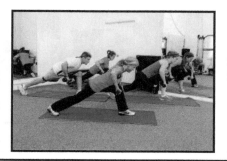

5. Bent Over Dumbbell Row in Lunge Position. Holding dumbbells in hand, bend over from the waist while in front lunge position, perform dumbbell rows by lowering weights to the floor and pulling them back up (as if starting a lawn mower).

6. Tricep Dip. Place hands at the edge of your seat and lower your body to the floor, using your arms to raise yourself back up. Be sure to keep your body close to seat/chair and squeeze your arms at the top of the move.

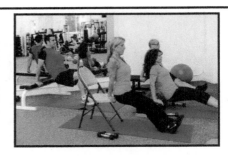

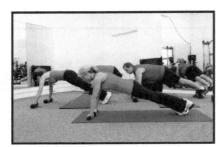

7. Pushups. Lay down face first on floor and hands next to chest. Push yourself up until body parallel with floor. Keep your body straight and core tight.

8. Lying Rear Fly. Lying face down with dumbbells in hands out to side. Raise dumbbells back in back as if you were "reverse flying."

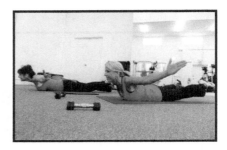

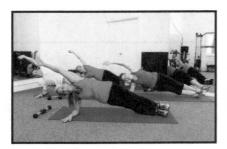

9. Side Core Raise. Lying on your side on your elbows, lift your body off floor using your core. Too hard? Use an arm or leg to help at first.

10. Plank. Lie face first on floor, body straight. Come up on elbows and toes using abs to lift. Hold as long as can, aiming for 1 minute.

You can order DVDs and download videos at lynfit.com

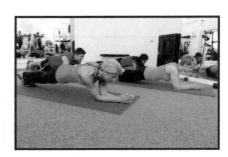

POSTURE POWER

They say the camera adds 10 pounds to your appearance. Proper posture takes those pounds away. Try it. When you stand your straightest you pull in your gut and use muscles you wouldn't be using otherwise. You look slimmer—but you're also burning more calories, strengthening your muscles, and breathing better.

When was the last time you heard someone tell you to stand up straight? To stop slouching in your chair? Poor posture is to blame for most back and neck pain—not to mention chronic joint pain. Posture is something you don't hear much about, but good posture is one of the most underutilized solutions that can change everything for you.

I have seen more people get in shape only to not look any better or different because they worked out with bad posture and made theirs worse. Did you know that the average person overworks their biceps, abs, and legs in workouts? These muscles pull you forward and the butt, hamstrings, triceps, and back keep you straight. Strengthening these muscles is the key to correcting the slumped posture that brings on pain.

> **GOT BACK PAIN? A WEAK CORE IS TO BLAME.**

Just about every client I know who experiences back and neck pain usually tucks her pelvis and tightens her glutes (butt), hyperextends her knees, turns her feet out, rounds the upper back, and sticks her neck out. Maybe you do all of these things, and most overweight people do all of them because their bodies adapt to carrying the load. But just because a body adapts does not mean it's a good idea. So what's so bad about doing these?

Butt tucking, also known as tucking your pelvis under, puts your whole body out of alignment and causes sway back, making your butt look flat and sloping your shoulders. This creates a domino effect from your head to your toes: Tucking your pelvis forces your feet and legs to rotate out, which in turn triggers low back and hip pain. This type of slouch also puts more pressure on your feet than they can handle as they are not designed to carry the load, potentially leading to flat feet and or plantar fasciitis. But hold on, it doesn't stop there.

When feet are not aligned, your knees take a beating and your tucked pelvis flattens the lumbar spine, removing the natural curve of the lower back. We need this natural curve for balance so we don't fall backwards. This is why we round our backs forward and stick our necks out—it's your body's way to adjust so you don't fall backwards.

LOOK LEANER

You can stand straighter. Get in front of a mirror and stand like this: Start off as if God has a string attached to the top of your chest and is lifting you up—this is better for posture than a

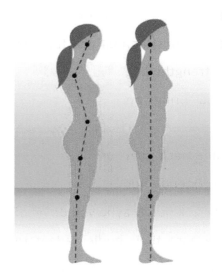

string to your head. Take a deep breath and exhale hard, releasing all your stress you're holding in your body.

1) Relax your shoulders and keep them pushed down and back
2) Be sure your ears, shoulders and hips, knees, and ankles all line up vertically
3) Pull your chin back so your head isn't out in front (this helps rid turkey neck)
4) Keep your pelvic neutral vs. tucked under or arched back (neutral), glutes relaxed. Remember you want a straight line.
5) Feet should be hip-distance apart and toes facing forward.

That's your starting point. Don't worry if you feeling overwhelmed; it may very well be a sign that you need this big time if normal posture feels so hard to you. Remember that imaginary golf ball? I always tell my clients to squeeze that imaginary golf ball—in the glutes for men, the pelvic floor (like Kegel exercises) for women. This really helps teach your body's core (abs) how to do its job. Anytime you feel back pain pull in your stomach, go through the quick and easy steps listed above, and it may just disappear.

Sitting posture is the same except your legs should not be crossed and you need to get up every 20 minutes and move or your discs slam together and cement in place. Not good. That's why drinking lots of water helps pain and lubricates your joints so they glide easily. This will also ensure that you get up every 20 minutes—you'll have to pee and that's good thing on both accounts. Also, be sure to have the right seat. I like a stool that I straddle so I actively sit and do not slump. If your chair allows you to slump, get rid of it and sit on a bar stool; you'll have less back pain because your core works (that's its job), not your joints. The core has incredible endurance when strengthened and used and will protect your joints.

> STAND TALL: YOU'LL STRENGTHEN YOUR MUSCLES, BREATHE BETTER, AND BURN MORE CALORIES.

Old habits die hard so if you are a leg crosser like me, switch legs every hour when you sit. Also switch if you tend to stand on one leg (put all your weight on one side). Standing with one leg supporting most of your weight throws your pelvis out of alignment and leaves you unbalanced.

STRETCHING TO THE HEAVENS

Remember the old childhood song "Head, Shoulders, Knees, and Toes" and how you'd touch each body part as you sang? Can you still do that? Can you touch *your* toes? If you want better moving muscles, you have to stretch—and not just the kind you do when you have a big yawn. As you age, your muscles tighten and movement can become painful. Stretching helps increase the range of motion of your joints and improve your flexibility. It improves your posture and gives you better blood flow. Daily stretching is the secret to reducing soreness and tightness so you can keep walking and doing your metabolic workout. You'll find the more comprehensive Recovery Stretch on my DVD, but Lazy Man's Yoga works in a pinch.

Lazy Man's Yoga   Don't forget to breathe!

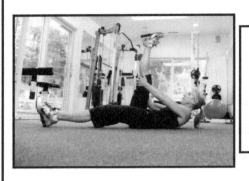

1. The Back Fixer (Lying 90-Degree Stretch). Life flat on your back and bring your leg straight to 90 degrees. Repeat other side.

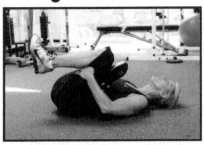

4. The Butt Stretch/Hip Opener. On back, bend leg at 90-degrees angle and place ankle of opposite foot in front of knee and pull knee back to feel stretch in butt and hips. Repeat other side.

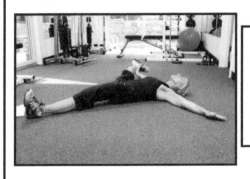

2. Lying Inner Thigh Stretch. Lying flat on back and stretch leg as far away from body as possible. Keep leg as straight as possible. Repeat other side.

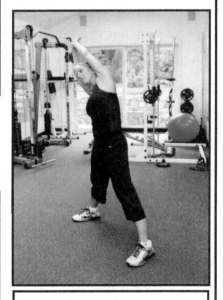

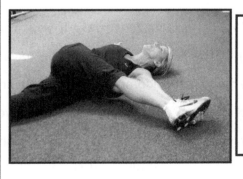

3. Lying Outer Thigh Stretch. Lying flat on back bring leg over and across your body (left leg crosses over right and out to left side).Keep leg as straight as possible.

5. Stretch Everything Out Stretch. Catch your breath. Raise arms above head and gently lean to each side, holding stretch 8 to 10 seconds.

I developed it after helping countless people who turned to me for workouts after injuring themselves through either over-exercise or other means. All my moves are done lying on your back using your core muscles to keep your body grounded on the floor. Breathing is very important to stretching, and it's vital that you exhale often. Breathing changes everything when it comes to stretching: It sends messages to your muscles that they should relax and let go of stress.

Not only will stretching give you better looking muscles, but it can help with joint pain as well. Pain, no matter what the cause or your age, is your body's way of letting you know it's out of balance. Pain is a symptom that something is wrong; it's an alarm saying, "De-stress, relax". Your body is telling you that you need to move. I always tell my clients, "If you rest, you'll rust". Exercise keeps your body limber and increases circulation all over, which delivers the nutrients your body needs to heal. Exercise also removes toxins, making it critical when it comes time to keeping your body in working order so that we feel good. And I know from my own personal experience that when I feel good I eat better.

Remember, you can always stretch on those days when you're not feeling very well. Our joints are designed like bladders and they need to be emptied in order to feel better. Have you ever noticed that you always feel better when you exercise and your aches and pains go away? There really is no excuse not to exercise. If you're short on time do 15 minutes of the DVD in the morning and the other 15 after work.

Tight muscles are a symptom of an over-stressed body that could be prone to injury. Best way to avoid this? Stretch. The wear and tear of obsessive exercising, doing the wrong exercise, or doing the right exercise the wrong way can be alleviated by stretching. After all, workouts are supposed to make you feel better, not worse. Stress less, eat less.

Seven

METABOLISM MIND GAMES

One of my favorite saying is *where your head goes, your body follows*. I believe your thoughts determine your outcomes because they guide you, powering your decisions right from the start. Your thoughts point you in certain directions that ultimately determine your end results; they create your attitudes and perspectives; and they also affect your relationships—specifically with your own body. Your thoughts determine how productive the weight loss, the transformation, will be and they influence every decision you need to make.

I realize looking back at my own background, during my time participating and helping in Dr. Hatfield's study, that I wasn't successful at losing weight because deep down I really

didn't believe it was going to happen for me. I never 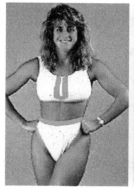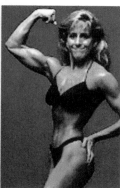 even tried to do what needed to be done, complaining that a certain diet didn't work for me or a particular workout didn't give me the results I wanted because it *wouldn't*. I believed what I was telling myself, I couldn't change, and my body simply agreed with me by staying fat. And even when some transformation happened, I couldn't see any physical changes because I was so buried in negative feelings about my body.

I struggled, hated my body, and wanted to change it so badly I could taste it. While crying about how miserable I was, I continued to eat all the wrong foods—the foods that were keeping me fat and slowing down my metabolism. I would exercise on and off, some days like a fiend, others not at all. And when it came to keeping a food and exercise journal, as we were all required to do for the study, I told myself and the other participants I was eating perfectly and exercising.

I truly believed I was eating healthy and exercising correctly. This is also known as a sincere lie: you believe what you tell yourself, regardless of its actual validity. For the study, I would literally sit in front of Dr. Hatfield's office and fill in my food/exercise journal with what he wanted to see, what he expected me to do. And when weigh-in time came, anxiety would set in and I would find myself coming up with any and every excuse as to why the scale didn't budge. It was stress; it was my period; of course I was following the plan and couldn't imagine why I wasn't losing weight. Sound a little familiar? I cannot believe I did that then. It seems comical now, but it sure wasn't at the time.

Why tell you this embarrassing story? Because every day I get thousands of emails saying something very similar. "I'm doing everything right and I'm still not losing." My first response is to ask for a glimpse of this "perfect" food journal. The food journal reveals all; and often it's filled with foods that slow the metabolism and cause weight gain—even the so-called healthy ones. There's bacon, whole eggs, whole-grain, organic bread, gluten-free pasta, avocadoes, nuts, yogurt, and cheese. Often I see my LynFit Complete Protein Shake made with fruit, juice, and soy, almond, rice, and even cow's milk. Not helpful if you are trying to *lose* weight. Others add a protein shake to an already fattening and carbohydrate-filled breakfast instead of having just the shake for breakfast, as intended. No wonder the calories add up.

Then there's the, "I'm-doing-Pilates/yoga/insert-your-favorite-workout-all-the-time-and-not-seeing-any-results", complaint. *The Metabolism Solution* is specific in which metabolic exercises to do. Doing an hour on the Stairmaster and then coming home from the gym famished is overworking. Do you have two or more hours a day to exercise? I don't.

We are human and far from perfect. It can be hard to stick to a food plan and hard to get the exercise in. *The Metabolism Solution* takes this into account. Forgive yourself for not being perfect. No one is. *The Metabolism Solution* is guaranteed to work every time if you follow the plan and eat accordingly. It is so effective, and here's a little secret I probably shouldn't tell you, that you will lose weight even if you do not exercise. Do not let "I don't have time to exercise" be your mantra. Don't get stuck thinking only about what you cannot do—think about what you can. Miracles happen in can's.

TURNING NEGATIVITY INTO POSSIBILITY

Do you think you're a glass half-full or glass half-empty kind of person? Do you let past mistakes drive you? Do you forever see yourself as the label an abusive person branded you with? Perhaps an early childhood experience has scarred you and influenced you in more ways than you realize? Have you ever asked yourself what your weight gain represents?

> FAKE IT UNTIL YOU MAKE IT—IT WORKS IF YOU WORK AT IT.

The answer may surprise you.

You have to choose to put the past behind you and move forward. I come from a divorced household with two alcoholic parents. If there were a Dysfunctional Family Olympics, we could have won the gold medal. I get how hurt feels; it is so hard to find faith and acceptance when bad things happen, but it's a choice you need to make. You have to trade your negative attitude for a positive one and believe you can be happy and healthy. But you have to decide to do so first. Dwelling on the pain keeps you in pain. When you complain, you'll remain.

If you can move on from it, you can change your life. You don't need to be angry to heal, and you don't resolve resentments with anger. Anger keeps you stuck where you are. Same unfulfilled job, same unappreciative spouse, same number on the scale. It's so easy to feed anger and resentment. You eat to ease the pain, then you gain weight and that causes more pain. So you eat again. You initial solution to pain is now the problem.

A key perhaps, is to live in the present, to feel gratitude for every God-given day, to feel hope that tomorrow is a new chance to try again. Once you have set your mind to let go of anger and resentment, stick to it and say the words of possibility every day: *I Can*. Start right now, turn your negativity into possibility. It isn't easy, so fake it until you make it—it works If you work at it. Don't keep repeating "It will never happen for me" again. It is up to

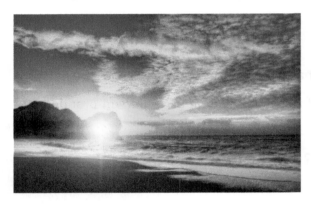

you. There are no excuses. Start now: Put all of your energy into the doing and you'll get results faster than you ever have. Discipline comes from the doing, and motivation follows.

Letting go of anger and resentments removes the #1 obstacle in the way of you leading the life God has in store for you. If you believe you will achieve, and where there is a will there is always a way. Stop using and believing in the words *I can't*. Working with other professional trainers and celebrities like Martha Stewart has taught me that we all wake up with the same amount of time in a day and we all have the same choices. It's simply a question of whether we will make the right choices. With the information found here on weight loss and how to supplement safely, nothing is standing in your way. Take it one day at a time, one meal at a time, one workout at a time. You cannot take a day "off" while trying to lose weight because it will stop your momentum and slow your metabolism. You don't need to trigger bad eating that isn't helpful in the long run. Change your thoughts and you'll change your body. Quitting is not an option because failure is not an option. This has worked for me for over 25 years.

It also helps me to stay positive by surrounding myself with positive people. I had the self-pity parties that would paralyze me and stop me from making the changes needed to get control of my weight. Misery loves company and you can always find those who will agree with you, the over-eaters and under-exercisers, those that will support your negativity. Change isn't necessarily easy; surround yourself with people who have the same goals as you do so you can inspire and support each other. Find those who think it and do it. Find that ability in each other.

You don't need more people around you to help you eat the wrong things or keep you from the gym. It's time to find a workout buddy and see if your friends will eat healthy and forego desserts with you. Look around and think out of the box here; the best partners may be the most unsuspecting. Family members often mean well, but they are often the ones to teach us wrong eating and negative thinking.

Look for people at work or others who have the same goal in mind and create an accountability relationship where you each let the other know when you need help getting back on track with your food or exercise. Allow them to be firm to get you back on track by not letting you give any excuses. There isn't any reason why you shouldn't be taking care of your body by eating right and exercising. Eating clean, as with *The Metabolism Solution*, and exercising are the solution to almost every problem—from weight loss to achy joints to fibromyalgia to injuries to depression. No matter the issue, you cannot go wrong with exercise, eating your veggies, and lean protein.

EMOTIONAL EATING 101

You eat when happy, when sad, when bored. How do you know if you are an emotional eater? You know. Trust me. When I meet a new client, red flags immediately go up if he asks me during that very first session about eating a certain food or if he'll be able to go "off" the plan. Such questions tell me right away that this is someone looking for an excuse to cheat before he even begins. This is no judgment from me; it takes one to know one, and I am one of these people. Experience has taught me that a different approach and attitude makes all the difference. "I'll do whatever it takes," and "I'll do it as long as it takes" are the words and thoughts to live by when striving for weight loss. Do you need that glass or two of wine every day? To treat yourself with food? If you're saying "yes," then this is an indication that you use food to avoid feelings, or at least the uncomfortable ones. Those that answer "No," treat themselves to manicures, a movie, or new clothes—not a food reward. We're rewarded with food from childhood. (Ice cream after the school concert?) But this is a sure way to get fat and not the way to lose weight.

Those people who don't think of food as a comfort, who don't self-medicate with it, if you will, don't eat when stressed. They actually often *forget* to eat. If you look to food to make yourself feel better, you eat more.

Food addicts are emotional eaters. They live for food and think about it all day long compared to non-addicts, who need to remember to eat and don't spend the day thinking about their next "hit" as if food were a drug. Unfortunately, that is a perfect way to think of food—as a drug. Studies show that food, especially sugar, hit the same spot in our brain as drugs, hooking us and making us dependent on the very foods we should be avoiding. With a food addiction, you can never have just one of anything; the whole

> **ARE YOU A FOOD ADDICT?**
> 1. Can you never eat just one?
> 2. Do you pig out in private?
> 3. Do you ceaselessly go from one diet plan to another?
> 4. Do you eat to reward yourself? To make yourself feel better?
> 5. Do you feel depressed about your weight?

bag disappears in the seeming blink of an eye. Then what happens? You want more of that treat (potato chips, Yodels, doughnuts, bread—you name it) and will find yourself stocking up at the store and eating it every night.

It was not easy for me to get past this. I got "clean" with food by following a 12-step program. Overeaters Anonymous is a 12-step program that has the highest success rate in helping emotional overeating food addicts. It taught me that compulsive overeating is a three-fold disease: 1) Physical, sometimes you are just hardwired to want to eat more; 2) Mental, you are prone to short-circuit during times of stress; and 3) Spiritual, if you're not in a good relationship with God, you will struggle.

Nothing else that you might find on the internet or in a bookstore will help. All the information out there can paralyze you with misinformation and have you thinking you can't when you should be empowered by the information right here on these pages and ready to take control of your life.

YOUR RELATIONSHIP WITH YOURSELF DETERMINES YOUR OUTCOME

Your success rides completely on where your head is at. If you are a positive person who thinks positively, you will get positive results. Have faith in yourself and in God. But what if you are more like me and struggle with depression and self -doubt? It's not so easy to turn a negative attitude positive when you feel so awful.

To help turn the tide, you need to do these three things every day:

1) Exercise. Exercise helps release happy hormones, and we can never get enough of these.
2) Drink your shake daily. The right kind of protein provides the mood boost and nutrients needed to get your brain working at its best.
3) Supplement safely. Safe supplements replace lost nutrients that anxiety siphons nutrients from our bodies at an accelerated pace, creating the need for more.

YOUR ATTITUDE DETERMINES YOUR ALTITUDE

How do we become compulsive overeaters who can't stop? How to we get our food under control?

All behavior arises from a state of stress. Between the behavior and the stress is a primary emotion. Remember that there are only two primary emotions Love and Fear.

It is through the expression or processing (also known as feeling) and the understanding of the fear that we can calm the stress and dismiss the behavior.

I know exactly what you are thinking and where you are coming from. I have been there. Just remember that you have nothing to lose except weight, and if you try it and don't feel better, I'll refund your misery.

The proverbial light bulb turned on over my head when I was working with Bryan Post, one of the nation's leading child behavior experts. I learned that instead of feeling an emotion, I eat. I'd rather eat than let myself be stressed, mad, or angry. What I have had to learn and accept, and perhaps you do, too, is that all emotions are valid and should be felt. Emotions are simply emotions. It's not normal to be numb, to feel nothing, and when we overeat, we numb ourselves from pain, fear, anger, and more. Unfortunately, when we block these negative emotions, we block the positive ones as well. Husbands, kids, parents, and even pets avoid us unless we approach them from a peaceful, loving place. Have you ever noticed that? You push away the very things you want so desperately by stifling all emotions as opposed to when you are "food sober" and feel all feelings, work them through, and let them be. So when you are feeling stressed or upset, stop and think a moment before you open the refrigerator. Food is the problem not the solution, and it's keeping you from feeling the required feelings you are supposed to have daily.

> **WOULD YOU RATHER EAT THEN LET YOURSELF BE STRESSED, MAD, OR ANGRY?**

Using an addictive behavior to deal with stress is far too common. Shopping and even compulsive exercise are all "drugs" that can become just as addictive as food or alcohol. Eating is a way of running away from uncomfortable feelings. You can run, but you cannot hide from these uncomfortable emotions. They have a way of hunting you down—sometimes when you least expect it. It's not always easy, but it's best to look that fear in the eye and tell it that you are not afraid. You are on your side. I am on your side. Most of all, God is on your side. And for me, knowing that God is on *my* side has turned out to be all I need.

So how is your relationship with yourself? Not so good? Are you convinced you will love yourself if you just get a flat stomach, lean legs, or stop eating like a glutton? Real, lasting change occurs when we love ourselves. We have to love ourselves *first*.

HEAD HUNGER GAMES

Typically, there are two things that motivate people to do what needs to be done, to change: Love and Fear. When you act out of a place of love for yourself, you tend to want to eat healthfully; you exercise to nurture your body and to keep it in working order. You do the right thing, and not because you are afraid. Fear derails you. Fear makes you stressed and anxious, and these two factors are the #1 cause of overeating and binging. They are the reasons your hunger switch doesn't turn off.

Think about it for a second. Are you 25 pounds overweight? You know you are supposed to eat more vegetables, aiming for 10 servings and a little protein four times a day. Yet instead you think you're hungry and grab a crunchy snack or a sugar-filled food? Is your body physically hungry? Probably not. This is head hunger. And feeding this head hunger is what hurts the most.

Just as you reboot your metabolism, you can reboot how you react to your body's hunger signals and learn to eat when truly, physically hungry and stop when full. The Halt Principal is a simple test. Before you reach for that midmorning doughnut, Halt. Ask yourself:

Am I too **H**ungry?

Am I **A**ngry or **A**nxious?

Am I **L**onely?

Am I **T**ired?

Simple questions, right? Wrong. These are loaded questions, but it is totally possible to change your not-so-favorable habits into ones that boost your metabolism. How? Well, you can't avoid stress, but you can change how you deal with it. Stress hormones can add to belly fat, but did you know that stress can also help you lose weight at a faster rate? It's true.

We all know someone who has been under stress and seems to waste away, but eating when or because we are stressed is the true culprit when it comes to weight gain. Eating certain foods like crunchy carbs, yummy sweets, sauce-drenched staples like the #1 comfort food macaroni and cheese adds fat *fast*. When you add fat-filled food to your diet, your fat cells take it as a signal to store fat; on the other hand, when eating lean and clean proteins and vegetables does *not* cause fat to be stored under stressful conditions.

> WHEN YOU'RE STRESSED AND REACHING FOR THAT SUGARY SNACK, HIT THE PAUSE BUTTON. YOU WILL MAKE BETTER CHOICES BY NOT TRYING TO FEED THE STRESS TO MAKE IT GO AWAY AND YOU WON'T BE ADDING TO YOUR STRESS BECAUSE YOU FEEL GUILTY ABOUT WHAT YOU ATE.

Sometimes, you might find yourself feeling hungry all the time. Even after eating. If you are following *The Metabolism Solution*, you *are* eating enough to fill your body's gas tank. You will not starve, I promise you. This is head hunger taunting you. Being hungry is a good sign when on my plan: It means your metabolism is moving and you are burning fat. Don't give in.

If you are serious about losing weight and living a leaner lifestyle, this is what you need to do: Wait at least 5 minutes before eating when you are under stress and think you are hungry. Hit the pause button and wait. Pray. You will make better choices by not trying to feed the stress to make it go away and you won't be adding to your stress because you feel guilty about what you ate.

If someone had told me that my anxiety and fear were making me overeat, I could have spared myself 20 years of self-loathing and wrecked vacations. Looking back, I see now that I hated my body so much I never enjoyed anything—not swimming and especially not shopping. I never bought any new clothes because I was waiting until I reached that magic number on the scale. And once I reached my goal weight, I still did not get rid of my fat clothes because I didn't believe I could keep the weight off; I had too-good-to-be-true syndrome and was waiting for the other shoe to drop. This kind of stinking thinking is always present when you don't love yourself. When you love yourself, you want to take better care of your body.

> BY REPEATEDLY WRITING DOWN YOUR GOAL YOU CAN ENGRAVE IT INTO YOUR SUBCONSCIOUS, IN EFFECT, BRAINWASHING YOURSELF.

If you are serious about real results and permanent change, are you doing what needs to be done? Are you willing to do it? Can you change your thinking?

Change your thoughts and they become actions: What you think about is what you focus on and repeatedly do; if you think positively you will find yourself with positive action. Thinking negatively will stop you from staying on the plan, which works if you stay on the plan. Positive thinking can bring you peace—and that is always a good outcome. Surrender (fully) to the process. 100 percent.

Set your mind and keep it set; do not fall into paralysis by self-sabotaging analysis. There is so much misinformation available. Log off your computer, close the books, and focus on the fast results you will see when following *The Metabolism Solution*. It works 100 percent of the time if you do it.

Practice good habits daily and do not quit. Quitting is not an option and should not even be in your vocabulary anymore. Practice until you arrive at your dream weight and, once you arrive, you can decide then whether you choose to eat more freely—but you may find that it's just not worth it anymore because food has lost its power over you. Yes, it does happen.

> PERFECTION DOES NOT EXIST. 80 PERCENT IS AS PERFECT AS IT GETS. FOCUS ON PROGRESS INSTEAD.

Turn your fear into faith. Stop worrying and doubting and just do it. Any training and any small eating change is better than no change at all.

Fake it until you make it. When you wake up feeling defeated, you will fake it until you are over the negative thoughts. Repeat after me, "I am doing this. I can do this. I'm a lean, mean, fighting machine. I love me". My daily mantra was *Leaner, Stronger*. I repeated this over and over the entire time I was on the treadmill for 60 minutes a day and I also wrote it down 100 times every night.

Focus on progress not perfection. Perfection does not exist and you will fall down, so learn to forgive yourself. (You now love yourself—remember?—and we forgive people we love, including ourselves) Eighty percent is as perfect as it gets. Learn to love yourself no matter what. This is your primary goal.

> THE MOST IMPORTANT THING, and I cannot stress it enough, is learn to forgive yourself if you cheat. Of all the strategies in this book, this, most of all, is the one thing I want to leave you with. Be confident that you can make this change, so pick yourself up as quickly as possible when you, brush yourself off, and start fresh right now. Do not wait until tomorrow, Monday, or the New Year.
>
> Because you drink a protein shake every day, you offset those not-so-perfect calories we all eat from time to time. Remember, Complete Protein boosts your metabolism by 25 percent and blocks cortisol, the stress hormone, from rising. If you have been following the plan, your metabolism will be revved up and in high gear. *The Metabolism Solution* takes into account that there will be bad days. Simply get right back on the plan and continue like nothing happened.

Let go and let God. I believe in a higher power, and that higher power for me is God. He has you in the palm of His hand, always.

This cycle of eating because we feel bad and then feeling bad because we've eaten is a very slippery slope and is easy to spiral out of control. This is why we gain weight and continue to gain weight until we finally are sick and tired of being sick and tired.

A craving can be crushed by distracting yourself. Change your thought, move a muscle. Exercise is the best remedy. I need to keep busy to stop myself from thinking about food all day long. Now that I am thinking leanly, I turn to my list of to-do's before I open the refrigerator if I think I'm hungry after a meal. It has helped me to turn to my mile-long list of things to do instead of automatically turning to food. I try very hard to eat only when I am relatively happy and calm—not procrastinating, not upset, and not angry. Do not turn to food for comfort; it is the problem, not the solution.

Remember, no one is perfect and we can live lean 80 percent of the time, we're doing okay. When all else fails, have a legal binge. Eat from the list on page 110 only and allow yourself to have extra if need be. Giving yourself permission to binge, this will relieve stress and remove that urge.

This is the first day of the rest of your life. You will fall and you will learn to get up faster and forgive yourself. Focus on progress, not perfection.

Eight

GOD AND YOUR BOD

So what does God have to do with it? Everything! I could write a book on this subject alone. Every pain or ache we feel is rooted and intertwined with our emotional and spiritual health. What you believe—or don't believe—keeps you stuck where you are and holds you back from taking care of your health and losing weight. I have learned firsthand that not being able to lose weight has much deeper roots than a slow metabolism.

I have learned that I have to take care of myself, no matter what I'm feeling or experiencing. There is no excuse to not take care of yourself. Food and emotion used to go hand-in-hand for me. I had to learn to stop eating every time I felt an emotion I didn't like. I had to learn to accept and let go of old hurts and fresh wounds, perceived and actual, before I could get a handle on my eating habits and over-exercising. I needed to remember that I had God's love and faith in Him to guide me down the right path. Feelings are very powerful. Any medical doctor will agree that emotions can influence your health—and waistline. And faith has the greatest influence of all.

NOTHING IS MORE IMPORTANT THAN YOUR RELATIONSHIP WITH GOD

If you are serious about changing your body, you need to be serious about working on your relationship with God. I firmly believe that. Only with faith can you get rid of whatever baggage you are carrying or whatever behavior is holding you back. Repressing feelings, denying them, won't work. Change starts on the inside. This isn't just about feeling better, losing weight, getting fit. This is much deeper and far greater. This will turn your life around.

The *only* one you need to please is God.

The *only* approval you need is from God.

Listen *only* to what God has to say to you and about you, meditate on this every day:

> You are beautiful, precious, courageous, strong.
> You are smart, funny, and kind.
> You are unique and worthy of love and affection.
> You are healthy and vibrant and strong beyond earthly understanding.
> You are God's child and your worth surpasses all early things. He loves and adores you.
> It is because of Him that you have the ability to change your personal circumstance, to change the world.

Are you eating too much to mask a pain, to fill a hole in your heart? Are you happy? A therapist once asked me that particular question and I struggled to answer it. Outwardly I'm sure I appeared quite bubbly (I usually do). I had everything: I had reached my goal weight, I married a loving man and had two beautiful children, we had a nice house complete with four dogs, and my career was going in the direction I wanted. Yet inside I felt empty. And I couldn't explain why. I still had that emptiness and loneliness inside me from days that weren't so good.

YOU CAN'T BE FIT UNLESS YOU'RE SPIRITUALLY FIT

Again I put the question to you: Are you happy? Do you feel good every day? Are you satisfied with the life you are living? If you had to stop and think about your answer then you most likely are not happy. It is time to take off the limitations you have put on God and let Him in. Stop making excuses; trade your negative attitude for a positive one and open your mind as well as your heart. Believe you can be happy and healthy. Believe in faith. Make the choice to let God in.

The most important decision of your life is to place God in the center of it so that He can guide you to that happy place. Maybe you're already a believer and feel you do this. But has your work, family, or stress over health or work issues become the center of your thoughts every day? Are you obsessed with spending too much time in the gym or worrying about what you can and cannot eat? Is God in second place with you?

Becoming physically fit did not bring me happiness. I learned it was only half the battle. I needed to become spiritually fit as well. Likewise, becoming spiritually fit (did you know that 1 in 3 Christians is overweight?) is only half way to happiness without the physical component. During my days with Dr. Hatfield and his research studies, I worked with a wide range of bodybuilders and weightlifters. These strong men amazed me. They were able to do things that seemed to defy human understanding lifting several times their own body weight. They had faith—and not only in themselves. This group had faith in God. Being physically fit and taking care of the body God gave you is your responsibility; it is another way of worshiping Him. It is your duty and privilege to protect your health.

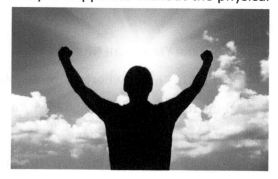

Coming to this understanding was one of the hardest journeys I've ever been on. I always considered myself a solid Christian woman, but after much, much contemplation I found that I had started to rely on food more than God. Food became my go-to source whenever anything good or bad happened. I was constantly asking myself, "Why shouldn't I eat this? Why can't I eat that?" I indulged myself. There's a word for you: indulgence. Look it up. It means "unrestrained action." My indulgence, unrestrained action, was eating. I was seeking pleasure in eating that I did not have in my life. This "pleasure" became unrestrained and a problem in and of itself. The more I ate to feel better, the more weight I gained. Thus my initial solution was now most definitely an additional problem. As I was, you need to be honest about how

LET GO AND LET GOD—OR BE DRAGGED

you rely on food. I was so lost in feeding my pain that I couldn't hear God's voice. God is here with arms open in love. Crave God the way you crave food. Don't let food become your god. Use God's presence to fill the void and emptiness that food now fills. Don't let food take God's place. Turn to God in times of stress and sadness, shout "Thank you, Jesus!" in times of happiness. Practice living a life full of gratitude and watch the miracles unfold that God has in store for you.

STRENGTHENING YOUR FAITH MUSCLES

A lack of faith. That is where many problems arise. When things aren't going your way, do you ever think to check in with God? Do you ever wonder that if maybe you had a little more faith you would be in a better place? Too many people spend too much time looking in the wrong direction searching for answers. Holding on to resentment is holding on to hopelessness, which is the opposite of faith. Faith is being hopeful, optimistic, and enthusiastic even in the worst situations. Faith is believing God will guide you and show you light in your darkest hour. You cannot be truly physically fit without being spiritually fit. I have no doubts. You are a spiritual being with human existence. The two cannot be separated. You are only as strong as your weakest muscle. Do your faith muscles support you?

> FEAR LOOKS DOWN AND WORRY LOOKS AROUND, BUT FAITH ALWAYS LOOKS UP.

Every issue you face, from health to financial ones, can be helped by developing a closer relationship with God. Your belief system affects everything you do—including the foods you eat and the way you live your life. If you don't believe something will work, you won't even take the first step. Your beliefs affect every choice you make every day, including whether to take care of yourself or not.

I made the choice. I choose to see good in every situation, especially the worst ones. I have strengthened my faith muscles by reestablishing my relationship with God. Only then did I begin to lose weight. Faith gives me courage and lets me make changes. Think of it this way: Fear looks down and worry looks around, but Faith always looks up.

> **All things are possible through Christ who strengthens me!**
> —*Phillipians 4:13*

With strong faith muscles you can keep God in the center of all things and never let anything get in the way of your relationship with Him, including your health issues, weight gain, or daily problems. With God all things work out for good; making all things possible. Putting God first set me free and it can do the same for you. If you are living your life based on fear, then you are not leading with faith. As your faith muscles get stronger, you'll lead with faith and fear won't take you off course. Faith gives you clarity.

> **Hate causes a lot of problems in the world and it's never fixed even one.**
> —*Maya Angelou*

Think back to feelings and food as discussed in the previous chapter. Dysfunctional beliefs, weak spiritual muscles, cause you to be dysfunctional, i.e., not take care of yourself, and the pain gets fed over and over again. You do not need to be angry to heal; you do not resolve resentments with anger. Anger keeps you stuck where you are. It is a key culprit in weakening your faith muscles. If you are ready to heal and get healthy both physically and spiritually, you have to let go of your anger, say goodbye to resentments, and find your faith.

> GOD GRANT ME THE SERENITY TO ACCEPT THE THINGS I CANNOT CHANGE, THE COURAGE TO CHANGE THE THINGS THAT I CAN, AND THE WISDOM TO KNOW THE DIFFERENCE.

Meditation is the exercise needed to strengthen your faith muscles. You might think it different from prayer, you might not. Meditation is a contemplation or thought and reflecting on it. When you meditate on positive things such as God's promises, you will feel good. If you continue to obsess on your problems, you will feel bad and it will be harder to turn your thoughts around as God's voice gets dimmer. Finding faith is finding optimism, a belief that in God all things will work out; things happen for reasons you may not be able to understand, faith helps you get through it.

Faith brings clarity. Faith helps you accept the things you cannot change, but more importantly, faith gives you the wisdom to know the difference between what you need to accept and what you can change. Remember, acceptance is not resignation, acceptance is accepting what is real and not being resentful about it.

To begin to find this clarity, to strengthen your faith muscles, understand this:

God runs the show.
God calls the shots.
All we have to do is show up.
Don't give away God's power to a diagnosis, a divorce, or any other negative situation.
   Give it to God.
We are all God's children and He loves us all equally and unconditionally.

Think about it. There is always someone out there who is in your corner. You are never alone. Accept this. Use these words as a meditation.

Another thought to meditate on? What is God's role in your life? Do you realize the part He plays? Do you grasp how much He loves you? Listen to only what God has to say about you, and He thinks very highly of you. Regardless of who you think you are or how you feel, you are the child of the Most High God who is powerful, and strong. It is because of Him that you have the ability to change the world and your circumstances (all of them) forever.

God loves you and He adores you and He created you fearlessly and courageously so that you can go and strengthen your spiritual muscle and find that person who may be buried under 40 pounds of excess weight or under that diagnosis that is holding you down or any fear that has been paralyzing you and clouding your thinking. Tap into the God source and release that person you were created to be. It's your responsibility to set that person free.

Once you practice these meditation exercises you will begin to see His work in your life and you will begin to remove the obstacles that keep you from seeing God's Grace. You will strengthen your faith muscles.

> The only person you need to please is God. The only person's approval you ever need is God's.

Any other voices that are telling you bad things about yourself are nothing more than your spiritual muscles begging you to work them out. Go back to the basic meditations listed here over and over as many times as it takes or until you feel better or see the change you are waiting for.

> **Do you not know that your body is a temple of the Holy Spirit who is in you, whom you have from God, and that you are not your own? For you have been bought with a price. Therefore, glorify God in your body.**
> —1 Corinthians 6:19

For every problem God has a solution. Take it to God. Give everything to God: Worry about nothing and pray about everything. Prayer is heavenly intervention and gives God your permission for Him to step in. In order to be healthy spiritually we need to pray every day.

If you are stuck and just cannot lose weight or get out of your circumstances you need to ask yourself: What are you meditating on every day? Your own problems? Or our God's solutions? We all mediate every day without even knowing it. If you mediate on gratitude, you feel grateful; if you mediate on how bad your problems are, you'll always see your life through your problems and you won't be able to see clearly. Faith gives you clarity.

> GOD MADE YOU WONDERFUL. PSALM 139 SAYS YOU ARE WONDERFULLY AND FEARFULLY MADE. YOU ARE BEAUTIFUL AND LOVED, NO MATTER IF YOU'RE A SIZE ZERO OR A SIZE THIRTY. YOU ARE BEAUTIFUL JUST THE WAY YOU ARE. GOD LOVES YOU SO MUCH THAT HE DOESN'T WANT YOU TO STAY IN A PLACE OF DEFEAT.

The bottom line? Most people meditate on pain, which cause them to relive pain from

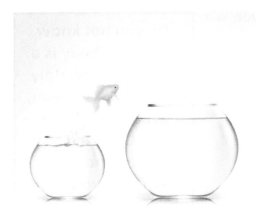

a very long time ago. Why do they—why do you—continue to feel pain that happened so long ago? Pain can serve a very productive purpose. Its appearance, physical and spiritual, alerts you to the need to address something and is actually productive. It tells us we need to address something and it applies to both physical and spiritual pain. Unfortunately, if you're faith muscles are not strong enough, the pain won't fulfill its productive role but drag you down. If you live your life based on fear, then you not leading with faith. When your own faith muscle gets stronger you'll lead in faith and fear won't take you off course.

What course of action is open to you when you know you have faith muscles weakened by anger and resentment? Finding the truth about yourself. Listening to truths about yourself is not easy; it's downright hard. But to process the feelings and ultimately feel

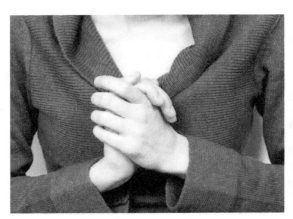

God's love, you need to. You are not a bad person because your worry about everything or live in fear.

Now that you've done the basics with meditation, you can further strengthen your faith muscles with prayer. Spend quiet time with God every day. I know how difficult this can be in our busy world so here is a way to begin praying:

Quiet Time with God to Strengthen Your Faith Muscles

- *Be alone with God and willingly bring your entire self to him.*
- *Allow your mind to settle so your soul can emerge. Breathe in and out slowly and focus on your breath until you feel relaxed.*
- *Recognize that God is as near as your own breath. IF you are holding your breath or not exhaling, you are blocking God from entering.*
- *Hear God calling: "Come away with me to rest a while"*
- *Is there anything that is hurting you or that you're struggling with these days? What is it that you have been holding onto? Have you lost your perspective?*
- *Allow it to come to the surface, whether it seems big or small—God will guide you through it so you can relax.*
- *Whatever feelings rise to the surface (for some you will need time to become aware of), know that you are not alone. You're in the presence of the one who loves you.*
- *Trust your deepest feelings and thoughts to God.*
- *Is there something you're feeling stressed about lately? Is something bothering you physically or spiritually? Ask God what you need to see. Perhaps you are grateful and need to express gratitude? God loves thankfulness.*
- *Let it rise to the surface without judging and bask in the goodness of God toward you instead of letting your feeling override God's grace.*
- *When your quite time with God is over, carry the sense of being alone with God with you into your day in everything you do.*
- *When you begin to feel stressed repeat as often as needed.*

FOR BEST RESULTS: Practice these steps three times each day. Find a quiet place where you will not be interrupted. I suggest doing your spiritual workout first thing in the morning before anyone is up. That's what Jesus did.

Remember to focus on your breathing and breathe in and out as slowly as you can. If you are harried and stressed, gently slow your breathing down by focusing on your breathing and inhaling deeply and exhaling as slowly as possible in order to relax your body. Tell your body to wilt as you slowly exhale (especially the tense-tight muscles) so you're totally relaxed and open to receiving. Take your time and take as many deep "cleansing" breathes as you need until you feel relaxed. A cleansing breath is when you exhale hard and visualize any ache or pain you have leaving your body as well as any negative thoughts. Each time you exhale visualize all of you stress leaving and God taking it to handle for you

When my mind races I start with the serenity prayer: God Grant me the serenity to accept things I cannot change, the courage to change the things that I can, and the wisdom to know the difference.

I struggle with learning how to love, how to forgive, and how to nurture myself. I never miss a weight workout or a serving of broccoli anymore, but sometimes I miss my quiet prayer or meditation. I miss God's voice because I cannot hear it when I'm moving at 100 miles an hour. I need to be slowed down enough to hear His voice, and if I'm in a loving place with myself, I can receive his help. Did you follow that? I am not always in a loving place with myself and that's why I don't eat clean or take care of my body by working out. Not being in a loving place with myself more importantly means that I am not going to be open to receiving God's healing. If I don't love myself, I won't feel that I am worthy, and if I don't believe I am worthy, I most likely will never take the proper steps to reach my goals. See how belief, faith, has everything to do with our outcomes? If you are walking around 30, 50, or 100 pounds or more overweight, you are letting the world know that you don't love yourself and because of that do not take care of yourself inside and out.

> ...Take time and trouble to keep yourself spiritually fit. Bodily fitness has limited value, but spiritual fitness is of unlimited value, for it holds promise both for this present life and for the life to come.
> —1 Tim 4:7-8 (Phi)

> **THE 10-SECOND SPIRITUAL DETOX**
> Ask yourself if there is one thing, event, or person that you can think of that makes your blood boil. Give yourself 10 seconds to think about it and then stop. What came up? Unfortunately this mediation exercise may not leave you relaxed upon completion, but it will ultimately help you regain your faith. It's important to do it until you can figure out what or who you need to forgive and process those feelings so you can be free from the pain.

Are you ready to radically transform your life not just your body? Remove any and all limitations you have placed on GOD and allow him to do His work as He wants to bless you with the desires of your hearts no matter what they are (especially the physical ones). This Spiritual leaner lifestyle also comes with a side effect of abundant peace, joy, and a love that surrounds you, making you feel whole, complete, and loved like you've never experienced before.

If you're ready you can trade all of your stress, anxiety and health issues simply by following the rules already set in the Bible; this book simply helps you with recipes and exercises that bring God closer to you so you can actually hear His voice and see where it is He is trying to lead you. Did you know that crazy lifestyles (including over-volunteering at a church that we all fall into) can make it difficult to really hear what it is God wants you to hear? Being intimately in touch with God brings an emotional sobriety to your life. When you aren't eating right or working out or resting enough or spending enough time alone so God can talk to you directly, you are "emotionally drunk" and cannot hear God's voice the way you need to in order to make necessary physical, mental, or lifestyle changes that heal your life and not just your body. Do the 10-Second Spiritual Detox Exercise described previously. It's not easy (to say the least) facing unpleasant feelings. And food, especially sugar and unhealthy foods which give you a "sugar high," can stifle your feelings. Try eating clean for a week and then doing this meditation. it holds the secret to your success.

CLEANSING FOR CLARITY

Sometimes no matter how hard you might try to focus on the good things, all you can see is the bad. Fasting can really help with this. All religions fast and some have had the tradition to do so for centuries. Fasting is more than just not eating meat on Fridays. Fasting is a way to leave behind the physical and focus on the spiritual and become closer to

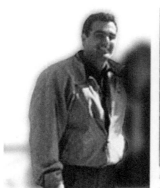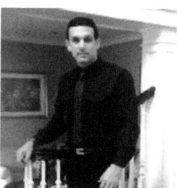

Pastor Frank – Lost 67 Pounds!

Real People. Real Results.
While all people are different and individual results will vary, these photos are of LynFit's customers' actual experience.

God. My pastor, Frank Santora, put it this way: "Fasting empowers us to progress rapidly

> **IF YOU WANNA GET RID OF THE PUDGE, YOU GOTTA LET GO OF THE GRUDGE. FASTING AND GIVING IT TO GOD ARE THE SOLUTION.**

toward the heart of God. When we deny our flesh, our spirit becomes more sensitive to the voice of God. Anytime we deny our flesh, our spirit antenna becomes more sensitive to God's voice."

His fellow Pastor, Rich Perez, added, "Fasting allows us to remove the mindset of self-centeredness and allows us to become totally dependent on our Creator God rather than our own resources and self. It removes our dependency from all things that block our sensitivity to our Spirit."

I fly a lot for various appearances, and on one flight was lucky enough to sit next to a Rabbi with whom I had a wonderful discussion about God. We touched upon fasting, and Rabbi Shmuly concurred with the two pastors. "There is no need to eat when we are focused on God. By fasting, we rise above the everyday and live on a higher spiritual plane. Fasting creates a euphoria that energizes us."

Jesus fasted to hear and understand God's voice and His directions for His life. So should we.

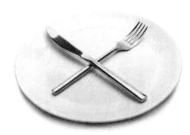

For me, fasting is a life-changing experience. At the beginning of my weight loss journey, I specifically fasted on the foods I was addicted to—carbohydrates, cheese, and processed foods. I stopped those instant-gratification food fixes. Instead of obsessing over what I ate, I was free to focus on life and what God wanted for me. Elements of this plan came to me at those times, and more importantly came my deeper feeling of God's love.

Moses fasted for 40 days. Jesus fasted for 40 days. Fasting helps bring us back to God, to family, to love. There is no instant gratification in fasting, there is only a deep and lasting satisfaction from a connection to God.

My decades of training and helping others reach their weight loss goals has taught me that people do better on a highly structured plan, even when fasting. And remember, fasting doesn't always have to be about food. You can fast from exercise if you're an over-exerciser (just walk every day for health) and see things fall into proper perspective. *The Metabolism*

> **WDJD.** I LIVE BY THE SAYING "WHAT WOULD JESUS DO?" but have you ever wondered what Jesus did to keep himself fed and fit? What Did Jesus Do? Have you ever given a thought to how much and how far Jesus must have walked? Jesus worshipped by taking care of his body. We are supposed to imitate him. Do you?
>
> Yes, Jesus never had to worry about all the snack food choices we face today and he didn't have the convenience of automobiles. Foods were often simpler, cleaner. Physical labor and having to walk everywhere kept people fit. We can all become like Christ—by following the overall style of life He chose for Himself. Prayer, meditation on God's word, and fasting kept Jesus close to God. If we have faith in Christ, we must believe *He knew how to live.*
>
> Jesus ate from the earth. He ate vegetables and fish and small amounts of lean meats. Of course He ate figs and nuts and He sipped on wine (sipped is the point). He walked everywhere so He was conditioned. Jesus ate dinner early when the sun was going down and woke up early at sunrise. There is much more to learn from the Best Teacher That Ever Was than you think.
>
> When in doubt, ask yourself: What would Jesus do?

Solution has helped me not only lose weight and keep it off, but it has helped me stay directly connected to God. I hear His voice clearly without interference. When I fall off the fast, off my plan, all the anxiety and stinking thinking come back tenfold.

The Metabolism Solution provides you with a plan that includes intermittent fasting to rev up your metabolism (full-on fasting would slow your metabolism down) and not hurt your weight loss goals the way other fasts can. No, I don't propose you go without food and water for days at a time, but I do see great benefit in my 48-hour Metabolic-Boosting Fast (see page 77). When I've fallen off my plan and indulged in my favorite food guilty pleasure, had a special dinner night out where I didn't eat cleanly, or am feeling out of sorts with the world around me and need to reconnect with God, a fast gets me back on track.

Any situation can be helped If you believe it can be. So why don't you believe you can lose weight? Are you lacking confidence? Worried? Worry is a lack of faith in God; replace your worry with faith in God. When struggling, with health or financial issues, with personal problems that never seem to end, it becomes increasingly harder to hear God's voice. It's not impossible to hear God, you just have to work harder. At least that's what I have personally found. I need God to inspire me to exercise and eat right every day.

Are you willing to do whatever it takes? Are you willing to do whatever needs to be done as long as it takes? Your body is not your god. Your scale is not your god. Food is not your god. See God the way you seek a good meat and you'll never be hungry again.

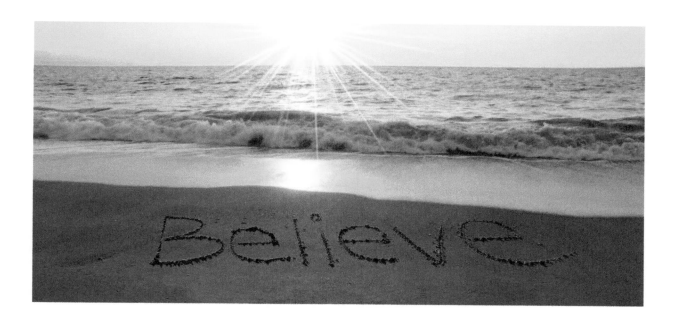

If there was a red button that you could push that would make losing weight and getting in shape faster and easier, would you push it? You just did by reading this book.

The Metabolism Solution is theanswer to your weight loss problems.

Are you ready for life-changing radical transformations? All you have to lose is weight. Unlike other programs *The Metabolism Solution* is guaranteed to work if you work it—or I'll gladly refund your misery. You have to believe or you'll never even start. You have what it takes. God is on your side, so how you can you fail? Get ready for the new, leaner, happier, and more vibrant you.

Start today!

Nine

IRRESISTIBLY DELICIOUS THERMOGENIC RECIPES

After 13 years with Martha Stewart, I've learned a thing or two about cooking. Anyone can cook with butter and oil. It's an art to create tasty dishes without them. Did you know that professional chefs practice a new recipe at least 10 times to get it just right? Practice until you get it right.

Now that you are armed with the knowledge of the thermogenic foods you need to eat for weight loss, wouldn't you like to prepare some mouth-watering meals using them? Here are the recipes to satisfy and de-fatify. Some of them may seem familiar as I've taken several

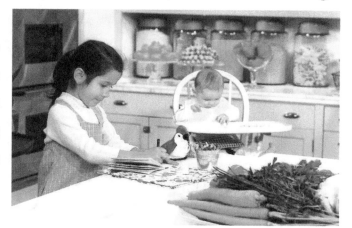

comfort-food-type dishes—and my childhood favorites—and remade them thermogenic-style. That doesn't mean these recipes are low on flavor. Each recipe is Weight Watchers-, Paleo-, and South Beach-friendly and, more importantly, meets *The Metabolism Solution* requirement: low-calorie, low-carb, very low-fat, low-sodium, and gluten-free, while packing in all the good stuff—fiber, protein, and beneficial nutrients to boost your metabolism. It's food so healthy even your doctor will approve. And the best part? It's absolutely delicious. Your family will think you took a cooking class—all that for under 300 calories a meal.

Use the foods, condiments, and spices on the list to make your favorite meals thermogenic. When you're pressed for time, search for store-bought ingredients with the lowest calories, fats, and carbs. Be careful when it comes to sugar, too; so many foods—especially sauces and dressings—are loaded with it. Sometimes you need to shop around until you find a store-bought brand that meets your weight-loss needs and tastes great.

CHICKEN AND TURKEY

Cooking lean protein is very different from preparing red or fatty meat. Because they are lower in fat, chicken and turkey can dry out quickly, and because they are also lower in sodium, you'll need to add additional spices to get that same flavor your taste buds are used to. You can always add water or broth (or a low-fat sauce) to any recipe to make it moister.

POPPA VINNIE'S TURKEY MEATBALLS

Minutes to Prepare: 20   ◆   Minutes to Cook: 40   ◆   Number of Servings: 6

I know every cook claims to make the best meatballs, but none compare to my grandfather Vinnie's. (Don't tell my mom) I've modified his original recipe, using turkey instead of beef and baking instead of frying to make it low-fat. You will not find a better leaner meatball. I enjoy these on top of a bed of broccoli along with a green salad. You can modify the recipe for turkey burgers as well.

1lb 97% lean ground turkey*
3 garlic cloves, minced
1/4 cup onion, finely chopped
1/4 cup parsley, chopped
1/2 teaspoon pepper
1/2 teaspoon oregano
2 egg whites, beaten
1/2 cup dry Italian seasoned
    breadcrumbs
1 tablespoon fennel seeds (optional)

Always sauté your onions and garlic first and then mix all the ingredients and shape into 30 meatballs approximately 1 inch across.

Place meatballs on a nonstick baking pan that's been lightly sprayed with olive oil and bake for 15 minutes. Turn them once and cook for another 25 minutes. Cooking times may vary-keep your eyes on these precious meatballs so they don't burn. You can always throw them into your sauce and cook them for the remainder.

*Use 97% lean ground turkey or stick to eating them once a week as the ground turkey meat bought in most supermarkets isn't lean enough and will SLOW your weight loss. Grind up your own turkey breast in a food processor to really keep it lean—it doesn't get better than that.

GAETANO'S CHICKEN SCARPIELLO

Minutes to Prepare: 10 to 15 ◆ Minutes to Cook: 10 to 15 ◆ Number of Servings: 4

This was my great Uncle Guy's (Gaetano's) family recipe. I make this in a flash and it appeals to all the senses. It tastes even better the next day—if you have any leftovers. Try it over a salad or make it the filling in lettuce tacos. You can cook this on a grill or in tinfoil for easier cleanup. You can also make this on a George Forman Grill by adding the peppers on top of the chicken breast. Want something different for cheat night? Make this with turkey sausage—but be sure to buy the leanest one you can find. I like Jennie-O's.

4 4 oz. to 5 oz. each chicken breasts
1 large red pepper sliced or 1 cup frozen
1 to 2 large onions sliced (frozen is fine)
1 small bottle of sliced hot cherry peppers and juice
1 tablespoon chopped garlic
olive oil spray

1 large green pepper sliced or 1 cup frozen
1 large yellow or orange pepper sliced
    or 1 cup frozen
1/2 teaspoon oregano
NoSalt and pepper to taste

Grill or broil chicken breast in oven or use precooked until partially cooked/warmed up. In a large skillet, sprayed with olive oil spray, sauté garlic, onions, peppers, oregano, NoSalt and pepper until partially cooked. (Add water or defatted chicken stock if you need more liquid so it doesn't get too dry.)

Cut chicken into bite-size pieces and combine with peppers and onions. Stir in hot peppers and juice, and continue to cook 10 to 15 minutes or until chicken is fork-tender—be careful not to overcook.

EASY ITALIAN PORTOBELLO CHICKEN WITH RED ONIONS

Minutes to Prepare: 5 ◆ Minutes to Cook: 12 ◆ Number of Servings: 1

It's no secret that I like to eat—and I like to eat a lot. I'm not proud of it, but luckily I have found a way to eat a lot and lose a lot, too. That's why this filling combo is good for you and your metabolism. I love chicken, but I just don't lose easily when I eat a lot of it. Mixing it with Portobello mushrooms is a good trick to fill you up while introducing different colors and textures to your diet. The color and texture of your food helps with overall meal satisfaction. Red onions with chicken and Portobello make this a metabolic-boosting, thermogenic combo. It's especially tasty over a big bowl of lettuce.

1/2 precooked sliced chicken breast
1/2 Red onion
balsamic vinegar

1 Portobello mushroom
olive oil spray
NoSalt and Pepper

Preheat oven to 425. Remove stem from mushroom cap, spray cap with olive oil and place stem side up on rimmed baking sheet or pan. Sprinkle lightly with No-Salt and pepper. Bake 15 minutes or until mushrooms are hot. Slice Portobello lengthwise into long slices.

While mushroom bakes, sauté onions in pan lightly sprayed with olive oil or on a George Foreman Grill.

When onion is glassy, add mushroom and chicken slices along with balsamic vinegar and heat all up while mixing together.

Be careful not to overcook. You can always add more balsamic vinegar or water if the balsamic vinegar evaporates.

GARLIC AND LIME CHICKEN BREAST

Minutes to Prepare: 10 to 15 ◆ Minutes to Cook: 25 to 30 ◆ Number of Servings: 4

Do you crave Mexican food but don't want to blow your diet? Eating this dish can save you thousands of calories and help you melt fat instead of gaining it. When we want Mexican flavor this is what my family eats. It's a great dish for company, too. I like to serve this with a chopped salad that's topped with a mixture of chopped cucumbers, sweet onions, and tomatoes chopped salsa-style and sprinkled with NoSalt and pepper, drizzled with a little bit of lime juice and 2 to 3 squirts of spray olive oil. This dish can be cooked in tinfoil or on the grill for easy cleanup. For a quick appetizer: Make extra salad topping to use as a dip for cucumber slices while you wait for dinner. Try the marinade for shrimp or as a dressing.

1/4 cup fresh or bottled lime juice
1 tablespoon olive oil
1/3 cup defatted chicken broth (look for gluten-, MSG-, and soy-free if possible)
1 tablespoon minced garlic (jar is fine)
4 approximately 5-oz. each boneless, skinless chicken breast halves (should shrink to 3 ounces after cooking); about 2 pounds total

Preheat oven to 400 degrees. In a large bowl whisk together lime juice, oil, broth, and garlic and season generously with NoSalt and pepper. Add chicken, turning to coat. If possible, marinate chicken, covered and chilled, turning once or twice, at least 2 hours and up to 1 day.

Remove chicken from marinade and arrange without crowding, in a shallow baking pan. Season with NoSalt and pepper and roast in oven until just cooked through, 25 minutes or less depending on your oven. Drizzle extra marinade and cover for moister chicken. Do not overcook.

Serve with tossed salad and green beans and baby roasted carrots.

GRANDMA MARY'S CHICKEN POTACCIO
(CHICKEN WITH RED WINE VINEGAR AND VEGETABLES)

Minutes to Prepare: 10 ◆ Minutes to cook: 20 ◆ Serves: 4

This is one of the best home-cooked chicken dishes ever. My Grandma prepared it and anything she made seemed like it was cooked with love and tasted dreamy. I can remember walking into her house and it smelled heavenly. Now you know how I learned that food was love. Be sure to make extra as this dish tastes even better the day after. This recipe works great and is much faster with small chicken cutlets or strips, shrimp, or fish—just adjust the cooking time and amount of spice as needed. Mangia!

4 medium boneless, skinless chicken breasts (cut up frying chicken fine for feeding your family)
2 tablespoon rosemary leaves
1 teaspoon olive oil
7 tablespoon chicken broth
10 garlic cloves (pre-peeled is fine)
1/2 cup red wine vinegar
NoSalt and pepper optional

In a large fry pan with a tight cover, heat olive oil and chicken broth. Add chicken, NoSalt and pepper, stirring often and cooking chicken to a nice golden brown. Add garlic, rosemary, and vinegar. Lower heat, cover, and let cook gently for 15 to 20 minutes.

When chicken is fork tender, remove cover, turn heat up to reduce liquid in pan. You can always add more water or chicken broth for more liquid and so chicken doesn't get dry. Keep in mind, there is no fat in this recipe so liquids may need to be added back in. Stir chicken pieces until well coated in pan juices.

Serve with sautéed escarole or green beans and, of course, always with a salad.

POPPA JIM'S CHICKEN TETRAZZINI

Minutes to Prepare: 10   ◆   Minutes to cook: 20 to 30   ◆   Serves: 4

My father loved to cook and Chicken Tetrazzini was one of his favorites Now that he is gone, I find myself wanting to make his favorites as a way to be close to him. This isn't his full-fat, metabolism-slowing recipe (he thought he was being healthy by eating chicken). I've swapped out those ingredients for leaner ones. This meal is for you, Pop.

4 medium boneless, skinless chicken breasts
2/3 cup or less of condensed evaporated skim milk (Omit for leaner meal)
1 teaspoon NoSalt
1/3 cup of sherry (optional)
Olive oil spray (optional)

2 tablespoon chopped garlic
1/2 cup grated Parmesan cheese
1 Lb. mushrooms thinly sliced (use an egg slicer for speed)
1 cup or more of fat-free chicken broth

Preheat oven to 400. Place chicken breast in pan with boiling water to cover. Add NoSalt and simmer covered for 15 to 20 minutes (checking often). Allow the chicken to cool in the broth.

Sauté mushrooms in fat-free chicken broth for 5 minutes. Cook garlic in 1 to 2 tablespoon of fat-free chicken broth or olive oil spray. Blend in remainder of broth, evaporated condensed skim milk, and sherry (if adding), stirring constantly over low heat until the sauce is smooth and thickens slightly.

Spray bottom of baking pan and layer it with chicken breast and cover with a layer of cream sauce and Parmesan cheese and mushrooms. Bake in oven until cheese is bubbling, 10 to 15 minutes. Serve with tossed salad with shredded carrots and mocked mashed potatoes.

Turkey Marsala

Minutes to Prepare: 10 ◆ Minutes to cook: 20 to 30 ◆ Serves: 4

4 boneless, skinless turkey breast,
    pounded to a uniform 1/4-inch thickness
1/2 tablespoon extra-virgin olive oil
1/4 cup chopped fresh parsley
minimal flour (optional)

8 oz. cremini mushrooms (stems trimmed), sliced
1/4 cup Marsala wine
1/4 cup low-fat, low-sodium chicken broth
salt and pepper to taste

Season each breast with a pinch of salt and pepper. Place the flour in a shallow bowl, add the turkey, and coat the pieces evenly, shaking off any excess flour.

Heat the olive oil on medium in a large nonstick pan or cast iron skillet. Add the turkey don't overcrowd the pan (do two batches if necessary) and cook for 3 to 4 minutes a side until the breasts are golden brown on the outside and cooked all the way through. Transfer them to a serving platter and keep warm.

Add more oil to the pan and add mushrooms and sauté until well browned.

Stir in the Marsala and broth, scraping up any browned bits stuck to bottom of pan. Cook until the liquid has reduced to about 1/2 cup. Season the sauce with salt and pepper and add the parsley. Pour the sauce over the chicken.

Good-For-You Chicken Stew

Minutes to Prepare: 10 ◆ Minutes to cook: 20 to 30 ◆ Serves: 4

I love this Chicken Stew. Fast and easy to prepare, it helps burn body fat. It's full of lean protein, vitamins, minerals, and fiber—giving your body all of the nutrients it needs to stay healthy and fit. Serve this chicken stew with a tossed salad for more oomph. Don't be afraid to adjust it to make it "your own." For instance, sometimes I make it with a marinara sauce. And it makes a great next-day grab-and-go lunch when you have extra.

1/2 teaspoon dried rosemary, crushed
1/4 teaspoon black pepper
2 tsp jarred minced garlic or fresh
1 Lb. skinless, boneless, chicken breast,
    cut into 1-inch pieces
3 1/2 cups torn spinach

1/2 teaspoon NoSalt (optional)
2 tsp olive oil
1/2 cup fat-free, low sodium, chicken broth
1 (15.5 oz.) can cannelloni beans or
    any other white bean rinsed and drained
1 (7 oz.) bottle roasted red bell peppers,
    drained and cut into 1/2-inch pieces

In a bowl, combine rosemary, NoSalt, black pepper, and chicken breast. Toss well.

Heat oil in a nonstick skillet over medium-high heat. Add chicken, sauté 3 minutes. Add garlic, sauté 1 minute.

Add broth, beans and peppers; bring to a boil. Reduce heat and simmer 10 minutes or until chicken is done. Stir in spinach, simmer 1 minute. Serve.

SKILLET TURKEY STEW

Minutes to Prepare: 10 ◆ Minutes to cook: 15 ◆ Serves: 4

This is a fast, easy, and lean yet hearty main dish that you can have on your table in minutes. Skillet Turkey Stew hits the spot and makes great use of leftovers. Serve it with a salad to complete the meal. For a change, you might want to add a drained can of garbanzo (chick peas) or white beans. Turkey is the leaner and more metabolism-boosting option than chicken, but there's no reason you couldn't use chicken or even fish if you want. Think out of the box.

1 tablespoon canola or olive oil (Need to make it leaner? Use spray oil.)
1 (14-oz.) can stewed tomatoes
1 green bell pepper, cut into chunks
3/4 cup picante sauce
1 teaspoon ground cumin

1 onion, chopped
1 onion, chopped
3 cups chunked cooked turkey or chicken
1 (8 oz.) can whole kernel corn, drained or peas—add your favorite
1/2 teaspoon salt

In a skillet, heat oil; add onion and cook until tender, about 3 minutes. Add tomatoes, breaking up large pieces with a wooden spoon.

Stir in remaining ingredients; simmer 10 minutes or until green pepper is crisp-tender.

SPICY SZECHUAN CHICKEN LETTUCE WRAPS

Minutes to Prepare: 15 ◆ Minutes to cook: 16 ◆ Serves: 6

This one is from my buddy Aaron McCargo, Jr., you may have seen him on Food Network. I helped him lighten this up for those days when you feel like eating a little cleaner: Took out the butter, reduced the oil, and swapped the chicken for turkey. Make it easy and just use McCargo's Signature Blend Seasoning (available at americanspice.com).

3 boneless skinless chicken breasts
2 carrots, shredded
3 stalks (1/2 cup) scallions
1 tablespoon Chinese five-spice powder
1/2 teaspoon sea salt
2 tablespoons grapeseed oil, for frying
1 head Bibb lettuce leaves

1/4 cup shredded daikon radish
1/4 cup bean sprouts
1/4 cup Szechuan sauce
1/4 teaspoon cayenne
1/4 teaspoon freshly ground black pepper
1 lemon, juiced

Split boneless chicken in half. If too thick, pound out to make thinner.

In a medium bowl, mix together radish, carrots, bean sprouts, and scallions. Add Szechuan sauce.

In a small bowl, mix together spices, cayenne, salt and pepper. Season chicken breasts lightly with rub. Cut the chicken into strips.

In a large skillet over high heat, add the grapeseed oil. Once hot, sear the chicken breasts for 4 minutes on each side. Add butter and lemon to pan and baste the chicken for another minute. Remove chicken to a platter to let cool. Once cooled, dice or shred the chicken.

Place a spoonful of the vegetable mixture and the shredded chicken onto each leaf of lettuce. Roll and serve.

BISTRO (BE LEAN) BUFFALO BURGERS WITH CARAMELIZED ONIONS

Minutes to Prepare: 5 to 10 ◆ Minutes to cook: 15 to 20 ◆ Serves: 4

There is nothing like the magic of seared beef-if you're a beef lover. I stopped eating meat for over 25 years to try to control my weight, and I must admit it wasn't easy to go back it. That is, until I found these buffalo burgers. Buffalo meat is just as lean as turkey and provides your body with all of the amino acids needed to keep you strong and lean. If you insist on red meat (once a week—no more), you need to look for buffalo burgers if you're serious about getting lean. I pile my buffalo burger on top of a huge mound of spinach greens and top with sautéed onions. McCargo's Signature Blend Seasoning in the onion topping turns it into a meltingly irresistible delicious meal, perfect for these hearty lean beef patties. Of course, the kids get cheese and bread, but I don't miss it. This also goes great with Lean Mean Green Beans Fabrizio-Style (p. 219). I like to buy my buffalo patties at Better than a Bistro (betterthanabistro.com), but you can also find ground buffalo in many supermarkets. This is so good.

4 Bistro Buffalo Burger patties or 1 Lb. ground buffalo
McCargo's Signature Blend Seasoning or your favorite
    spice

1 large onion, sliced
cooking spray
rolls (optional)

Spray pan with cooking oil and sauté onions sprinkled with McCargo's Signature Blend Seasoning or your favorite seasoning.

Form patties from beef if using ground buffalo.

Grill, broil, or fry patties. Be careful not to overcook them as they are very lean. IF you overcook add a little water to add moisture. Tope each burger with sautéed onion.

If Cooking Frozen Patties

Grilling: Adjust grill so that burger surfaces are 6 to 8 inches from coals. This gives even heat without too much intensity. If food gets too hot, raise grill away from heat.

Broiling: Preheat broiler. Top surface of burger should be 3 inches from heat. Rare, 8 minutes. Medium, 12 minutes. Well done, 20 minutes.

Frying: Preheat a heavy frying pan. When the pan is very hot brown burgers quickly on both sides. Do not cover pan. Lower heat and cook slowly until done. Turn a few times to desired doneness.

FISH AND SEAFOOD

The lighter and whiter the fish the better for your metabolism. Fish is good for weight loss because it's low in calories and fat and high in nutrients; it's the best source of Omega-3 fats. Simply put, the more fish you eat the faster and easier it will be to lose weight. Frankly, I like it because you get a bigger serving. You may have seen me talk about fish on TV, and eating more seafood is the best kept diet secret on the planet. I've taken special care to create recipes that even the fussiest teens will try. Set a goal to at least find one type of seafood you'll eat and focus on that. (And I did take sustainability into account when creating these recipes.) Also consider buying flash-frozen fish. It's more economical and you'll never run out of healthy food as long as your freezer is stocked with flash frozen seafood. I don't even bother with fresh anymore and rely on Vital Choice (vitalchoice.com) to deliver seafood to my doorstep.

SEXY SLIMMING SALMON

Minutes to Prepare: 5 ◆ Minutes to Cook: 10 ◆ Number of Servings: 4

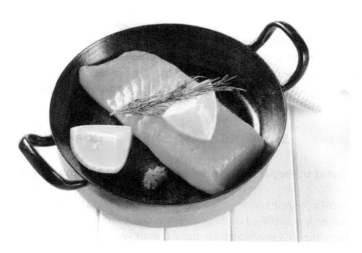

This recipe is one of the best when you're trying to cut calories because it's high in Omega-3 and therefore it takes a little longer to digest, which helps keep you fuller longer. My husband calls this "sexy salmon" because he knows I make this when I'm getting ready for a TV appearance or bathing suit season. Its exotic flavor will dazzle your family and I've never met anyone who didn't like it. This recipe is comforting in the winter but also grills quickly in foil. It goes great on top of a bed of spinach or baby greens along with string beans. Don't forget fresh raspberries or, better yet, raspberry sorbet for dessert.

1 tablespoon garlic powder
1/2 teaspoon salt
1 teaspoon sesame oil

1 tablespoon dried basil
4 (6 oz.) Alaskan salmon
4 lemon wedges

Stir together the garlic powder, basil, and salt in a small bowl; rub in equal amounts onto the salmon fillets.

Spray skillet with olive oil spray and place over medium heat; cook the salmon in the butter until browned and flaky, about 5 minutes per side. Serve each piece of salmon with a lemon wedge.

ITALIAN BAKED HALIBUT
(HALIBUT A LA SICILIANO)

Minutes to Prepare: 20 ◆ Minutes to Cook: 20 ◆ Number of Servings: 4

My family flips for this recipes—even the picky 13-year-old fish hater. It is incredibly delicious and not too hard to make. We like this dish paired with green beans and a salad or with ciambotta.

2 pounds of halibut (Pacific) or you can substitute
    tilapia, barramundi, or any other white fish
1 tablespoon dried basil or 2 tablespoon fresh
1 clove of garlic, crushed
salt and pepper

1 large onion sliced
1 can chopped stewed tomatoes
1 tablespoon dried parsley or 2 tablespoon fresh
dash of clam juice (red or white—your preference)
sliced black olives for garnish (optional)

Preheat oven to 450 degrees (375 for lighter fish). Wash fillets and dry with paper towels. Arrange in a single layer in 3x9 baking dish. Season with salt and pepper. Cover with onions, tomatoes, basil, parsley and garlic.

Moisten with a little bit of water or clam juice. Bake for 20 minutes or just until the fish separates easily when touched with a fork. Drain off most of the liquid before serving. Garnish with black olives

SLIMMING SEAFOOD STEW-CIOPPINO

Minutes to Prepare: 10 ◆ Minutes to Cook: 30 ◆ Number of Servings: 4

I learned about this particular cioppino from a Speedo model who had to stay very lean all year round and had lots of great ideas on how to feel satisfied and not wreck a waistline. This recipe has so much seafood in it that there's something for everyone. It's your stew, so make it your way. Keep what you like. You can keep it mild or spice it up by adding hot sauce and hot peppers. It's great served with a Caesar salad and bread or pasta for the carb eaters. When I have one of those I-gotta-eat days, this is now my go-to food because it's so delicious and oh-so-very satisfying. Cioppino is part of my traditional Christmas Eve dinner and it's so low in calories that I can spend those extra calories on dessert. Holidays unfortunately are not license-to-cheat days; our bodies still store fat regardless of the date. Try to focus on family and friends and less on the food—you'll enjoy the holidays even more.

1 medium onion, quartered
1 small lemon, sliced thin

6 to 8 garlic cloves minced
1 cup green onion chopped

1 cup red pepper chopped
1 teaspoon basil
1 tablespoon chopped parsley
1 tablespoon extra-virgin olive oil
1 (28 oz.) can crushed tomatoes in juice
1 Lb. of shrimp, cleaned
1 (8 oz.) bottle clam juice (optional)
1 Lb. skinless fillets of thick white-fleshed fish such
    as halibut, hake, or Pollack, cut into 2-inch chunks

1 teaspoon oregano
2 bay leaves
3 garlic cloves, smashed and peeled
1/8 teaspoon dried hot red-pepper flakes
1 1/2 cups water
1 Lb. cultivated mussels or clams or both
1 cup balsamic vinegar or full-bodied red
    wine such as zinfandel or Syrah
1 1/2 pounds of lobster tail cut up (optional)

Chop onion and garlic by hand or in food processor until coarse. Heat oil in a 5- to 6-quart heavy pot over medium-high heat and stir in all chopped vegetables, bay leaves, basil, red-pepper flakes, salt and pepper.

Cook covered over medium heat, stirring once or twice until vegetables begin to soften, about 4 minutes. Add tomatoes with their juice, water, wine, and clam juice (if used), lemon, and parsley and boil, covered, 20 minutes. Stir in seafood and cook, uncovered, until fish is just cooked through and mussels open wide approximately 4 to 6 minutes (discard any that remain unopened after 6 minutes). Discard bay leaves. Serve in bowls.

GAMBERI AL FORNO
(BAKED SHRIMP)

Minutes to Prepare: 5 ◆ Minutes to Cook: 20 ◆ Number of Servings: 2

Everyone loves shrimp—even fish haters. I love this dish for its simplicity and its sheer satisfaction. I make this at least once a week and especially when I have company. Pressed for time? Buy the shrimp already cleaned and cooked and sprinkle McCargo's Signature Blend Seasoning (available at americanspice.com) for a bold delicious flavor everyone will rave about. Keep a stash of flash-frozen shrimp in your freezer so you're never without fast, easy, and healthy meal options that won't break your diet. What's the best shrimp to buy? Look for domestic shrimp; pink Oregon is my favorite. In the winter this dish can be made in the oven and in the summer try it on the grill in tinfoil. It smells awesome on the grill and always lure a neighbor or two over asking what we are making because the garlic penetrates the whole block.

14 jumbo or 20 medium shrimp
2 to 3 cloves of garlic, chopped
olive oil spray
1/8 cup of white wine (optional)

juice from 1/2 lemon or substitute with store
    bought lemon juice
dash of paprika
salt and pepper (optional)

Preheat oven to 400 degrees. Peel and de-vein shrimp and place in a shallow baking dish sprayed with olive oil spray.

Sprinkle lemon juice and garlic over top of shrimp and spray with Olive oil spray. Bake for 20 minutes and or until cooked.

Add water or white wine to keep moist. Do not overcook. Check frequently. Garnish with paprika on top.

SCALLOPS PRIMAVERA

Minutes to Prepare: 10 ◆ Minutes to Cook: 20 ◆ Number of Servings: 4 to 5

I could live on this dish as I always feel very satisfied and full after I eat it—but never too full, if you know what I mean. Scallops make a typical dinner feel special and not diet-like at all. Scallops are one of the lowest calorie, lean proteins you can eat, and since you're having it with a truck load of veggies (no pasta in sight), you're saving yourself from having to burn off extra calories at the gym. You won't miss the pasta or butter in this dish—I guarantee it.

1 pound of scallops (fresh or flash frozen)
1/2 cup water
1/3 cup tomato paste (or you can use a 15 oz. can
    of crushed tomatoes with basil, oregano, and onion)
1 garlic clove minced
1/2 cup julienned carrots
1 cup broccoli florets
dash of pepper

3 tomatoes, peeled and chopped
2 tablespoon snipped fresh basil or 1 tablespoon
    crushed, dried basil
1 tablespoon fresh snipped parsley (or dried)
1 Lb. fresh asparagus
1 medium red bell pepper, sliced
1 cup sliced mushrooms
Parmesan cheese (optional)

Spray pan or wok with olive oil spray. Add garlic and cook for 1 minute (add some water if needed—do not let it burn).

Add carrots, broccoli, and peppers and cook for 1 minute. If scallops are frozen, add them with carrots and peppers.

Add scallops, mushrooms, tomatoes, basil, parsley, asparagus, and red pepper and continue cooking until done. Pour over bed of spinach and serve immediately. Garnish with Parmesan cheese if desired.

SLIM-QUICK TUNA BURGERS

Minutes to Prepare: 10 ◆ Minutes to Cook: 20 ◆ Number of Servings: 4

Even the fish-haters love these burgers. They are fast and easy to prepare and make losing weight tasty. I always suggest that you have canned tuna, salmon, or crab on hand at all times so when you run out of ideas or food so you always have a delicious—and good for your metabolism—backup available. You can make these burgers with ground turkey or fresh fish that you ground up yourself as well. Of course this recipe is leaner than most: no oil, mayonnaise, or egg yolks. Serve it on top of salad greens with green French fries.

2 5 to 6 oz. cans chunk light tuna, drained
1/4 cup finely chopped onion
1 egg white

1/4 cup chopped celery
1/2 cup medium salsa
spray oil—either olive or canola

Combine tuna, 1/4 cup salsa, celery, and onion in a medium bowl, breaking up any larger pieces of tuna until mixture is uniform and holds together.

Combine remaining 1/4 cup of salsa and egg white. Spray large nonstick skillet and place over medium heat.

Using a generous 1/3 cup each, form tuna mixture into four 2-inch burgers. Cook until heated through and golden brown, about 2 minutes per side.

Place on top of green salad and dress with your favorite salsa or mustard dressing for a big bang.

Too moist? Drain excess liquid. Too dry? Add more water or salsa. Make extra for lunch during the week or for a lean snack.

CRAB CAKES GET LEAN

Minutes to Prepare: 5 ♦ Minutes to Cook: 5 to 8 ♦ Number of Servings: 4

Fresh lump crab meat makes all of the difference in this recipe. But if you have to improvise, canned works. Crab meat makes a great burger patty at a barbecue when you want to eat healthy and treat yourself. I adore these all year long.

1 Lb. lump crab meat, drained and shell pieces removed or 2 to 3 6 oz. cans*
1/4 cup light mayo or for a leaner version use mild mustard
1 teaspoon prepared mustard
cooking spray
2 teaspoon Worcestershire sauce or horseradish for optional zing

1/3 cup finely chopped red bell pepper
1/3 cup finely chopped green bell pepper
1 teaspoon garlic powder
1/4 teaspoon paprika
3 large egg whites
4 lemon wedges

Preheat oven to broil. Combine everything but the lemon wedges and cooking spray in a medium bowl. Divide mixture into 4 equal portions, shaping each into 1-inch thick patty.

Place patties on baking dish coated with cooking spray. Broil 3 inches from heat for 8 to 10 minutes or until browned. Serve with lemon wedges over a bed of baby greens.

Keep your eye on these burgers as they are very lean and cook quickly. Grill them in foil on the grill to keep moist and together. If needed, you can add a tiny bit of breadcrumbs to tighten up the patties, but I like mine as clean as possible to leave room for dessert.

*Try them with canned salmon

GLAZED TUNA STEAKS WITH CRUNCHY CABBAGE

Minutes to Prepare: 7 ♦ Minutes to Cook: 10 to 12 ♦ Number of Servings: 4

Yum. And so easy to make. Great hot or cold and even better the next day. I crave this one to the point that I am always sneaking into the refrigerator to grab a bite. Thank God it's good for you. Tuna is high in Omega-3, Vitamin D, and Selenium—all of which are necessary for your body to burn stored fat. The soy sauce, typically a no-no for weight loss, is minimal so it doesn't do any damage. If you're in a hurry, substitute fat-free Asian dressing for the liquids.

1 tablespoon low-sodium soy sauce
(or use balsamic vinegar)
1 teaspoon garlic cloves, minced
(store-bought, prepackaged is fine)
1 cup shredded purple cabbage
sesame seeds (optional)

1 teaspoon mirin (optional; helps erase the fishy smell.
Rice wine for cooking may be substituted)
2 3 to 4 oz. each tuna steaks
6 cups shredded Savoy cabbage (ANY cabbage works!
If you're short on time, pick up some already
shredded from a salad bar.)

Combine 1/4 cup water, 1 tablespoon soy sauce (or balsamic vinegar), mirin (or rice cooking wine), and garlic in a small saucepan. Bring to a boil over medium-high heat. Stir together remaining tablespoon soy sauce, then stir into saucepan. Cook for 3 minutes over medium heat. Divide sauce into two separate bowls.

Place tuna in a skillet coated with cooking spray or a Teflon frying pan and add a little water so it stays moist and doesn't burn. Cook/poach tuna for 2 to 3 minutes per side depending on thickness.

In the saucepan add 1/2 of the sauce; add cabbage and sauté for a few minutes until desired tenderness is reached.

Meanwhile, place tuna in sprayed pan with remaining sauce. Lightly pan sear for a minute.

To serve, make a bed of cabbage and place tuna on top.

MOJITO-GRILLED FISH TACO

Minutes to Prepare: 5 ◆ Minutes to Cook: 14 ◆ Number of Servings: 4

This lean and light recipe is clean and can be used with any white fish or even chicken. Make extra. It is plate-licking good. I think this recipe tastes better with fresh vegetables because you can really taste the flavors each food brings to the dish. It's clean and mean you and you will be too. This dish goes well over a bed of shredded cabbage or with lime slaw (see Salads, p. 237) or can be eaten taco-style by using a lettuce leaf as your carb-free taco shell replacement.

1 pound firm white fish such as halibut, red snapper,
shrimp, scrod, cod, haddock, or tilapia—
they all work
1 teaspoon canola oil or canola oil spray
1/2 teaspoon salt substitute

2 tablespoons lime juice
2 tablespoons mint leaves
1 whole jalapeno chili pepper seeded and minced
(optional)

Combine marinade ingredients, stir well. Add fish to marinade. Refrigerate 20 to 30 minutes while making the rest of the meal, if possible, turning once. Remove fish from marinade and discard marinade.

Prepare grill for high-heat cooking. Place fish directly over heat; grill until firm, opaque and lightly browned. (I like to make mine in foil to keep it moist)

Not in the mood to grill? That's Okay. Make it in the oven, cooking for 4 to 7 minutes on each side. Cooking time may vary depending on fish and oven; keep an eye on it.

VEGETABLES

All of these recipes include fibrous, thermogenic veggies that serve as a great base for fat-free sauces (marinara) and proteins instead of pasta or starchy vegetables. My goal: Get you addicted to your own cooking to save you time and money and to help you lose that pound a day.

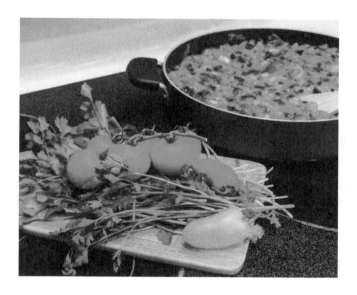

POPPA VINNIE'S CIAMBOTTA

Minutes to Prepare: 15 ◆ Minutes to Cook: 20 ◆ Number of Servings: 4

My grandfather used to make this hearty vegetable stew and it is one of my all-time favorite comfort foods. It evokes such wonderful unforgettable childhood memories for me. It's the Italian version of ratatouille, and everyone who tries it becomes addicted—even if they hate vegetables. "Ciambotta" means "tasteful and colorful." It's the dish that farm folks learned to perfect after the hardships of World War II when meat wasn't plentiful or affordable. I make Ciambotta every Sunday night. Fresh vegetables are best in this dish but frozen ones work in a pinch. Enjoy it as a side dish or as a main course by adding in shrimp, cubed chicken, or swordfish, or by mixing it together with egg whites.

1 large red bell pepper

3 plum tomatoes, chopped or 1 32 oz. can of
    chopped tomatoes with garlic, basil, and oregano

1 medium eggplant

handful fresh basil leaves

1 teaspoon olive oil

1 large green pepper

1 medium zucchini

1 10 oz. package mushrooms

1 large onion

3 minced garlic cloves

NoSalt & pepper to taste

Cut all vegetables into 1/4-inch pieces. Lightly salt eggplant pieces to draw out moisture and collapse their spongy texture. (It also helps them to not absorb all the oil)

Heat oil in a large skillet. Add onions, cooking until soft, then add peppers. Cook about 10 minutes on low heat. Add rest of vegetables including basil. Salt and pepper to taste.

Cook until all vegetables are soft, about 15 minutes.

BROCCOLI A LA PIZZOILA
(BROCCOLI SICILIAN STYLE)

Minutes to Prepare: 10 ◆ Minutes to Cook: 20 ◆ Number of Servings: 4

This is one of my personal favorites and, quite frankly, I could live on this every day of my life. The recipe says this serves 4, but I can eat the whole thing. Thank goodness more vegetables are always better when it comes to losing weight. To make a meal of it, I simply add shrimp, fish, or shredded chicken. When I need lots of filling comfort food I add water or an extra can of chopped tomatoes and turn it into stew.

1 large bunch of Broccoli
4 anchovy fillets, cut into pieces
1/2 teaspoon NoSalt or other salt substitute
or
1/2 teaspoon pepper
1 tablespoon chopped garlic or garlic powder to taste
1 tablespoon grated provolone cheese (optional)

1 large onion sliced
1 can chopped tomatoes with basil, oregano, and garlic
    (or you can use defatted or fat-free chicken broth
    water for steaming)
olive oil spray

Clean broccoli and cut into bite size pieces.

Spray bottom of pan with olive oil and place chopped onion, garlic, and one layer of broccoli. Add a sprinkle of cheese, NoSalt, and pepper and spray with olive oil until lightly covered.

Repeat layers until all broccoli used. Spray again with olive oil and add canned tomatoes. Cover pan and cook over low heat for 15 to 20 minutes until broccoli is tender.

BAKED ITALIAN CAULIFLOWER
(METABOLIC-BOOSTING MOCK MASHED POTATOES)

Minutes to Prepare: 10 ◆ Minutes to Cook: 20 ◆ Number of Servings: 6

We always called this one Grandma Matasko's Baked Italian Cauliflower and it is one of the best-tasting vegetables you'll ever eat. Every kid who comes to my house eats this up and always asks for more—despite the fact that their parents swear their kids won't eat vegetables.

1 large head cauliflower*
1/2 cup grated Parmesan cheese
NoSalt or salt substitute

1 tsp olive oil and olive oil spray
1 teaspoon garlic powder
1 tablespoon breadcrumbs (optional for top)

Wash and clean cauliflower, break into flowerets. Boil for 5 minutes in salt water until half done. Drain. Or you can microwave it or steam it on the stove top.

Spray bottom of pan with olive oil spray and arrange cauliflower on bottom.

Combine bread crumbs (if used) with grated Parmesan cheese and sprinkle over cauliflower. Season with pepper and garlic powder. Spray top to coat w/with olive oil spray.

Bake at 350 degrees for 15 to 20 minutes. If it becomes dry, add water to keep moist. Cooking times may vary depending on oven and keep in mind your cooking very lean which means no or less oils and fat so things cook faster and dry out quick making it necessary to add liquid back in.

*Double up the recipe and mash for Mocked Mashed Potatoes to boost metabolism anytime mashed potatoes are called for. No one will notice the difference if you don't tell them. Seconds allowed.

LEAN MEAN GREEN BEANS FABRIZIO-STYLE

Minutes to Prepare: 5 ◆ Minutes to Cook: 5 to 10 ◆ Number of Servings: 4 to 6

Every person I have ever worked with who hates vegetables loves green beans. My 13-year-old fussy eater calls these green French fries. They are a great finger food—even delicious cold. I make these green beans every single week to guarantee my kids eat their vegetables without my asking. Even with ketchup they're still healthier than French fries. They also serve as a great grab-and-go snack. Just prepack them in a plastic container so they're ready to go when you are.

1 Lb. fresh green beans (or frozen)
1 can chopped tomatoes with garlic, basil, and oregano
NoSalt and pepper

1 to 2 tablespoons chopped garlic (store bought works)
olive oil spray

If preparing fresh beans, cut off tips and remove any strings and break in half. Cook quickly in chopped tomatoes with their liquid until crisp and tender (do not overcook). Keep cover off to retain vibrant green color. Cool under running water to room temperature.

If preparing frozen follow package instructions. Or simply thaw if making cold.

Place cooked beans in serving bowl. Spray with olive oil and season with garlic, NoSalt, and pepper.

PASTA NOT!—CARROTS, ZUCCHINI, & SQUASH RIBBONS

Minutes to Prepare: 10 ◆ Minutes to Cook: 10 ◆ Number of Servings: 6

Do you ever wonder how you'll survive without pasta? I used to think that. What I've learned is that it wasn't the pasta I was addicted to but rather the sauces. Pasta is nothing more than a fattening, metabolic-slowing food that is highly over-rated. These recipes are all about finding tasty replacements for those metabolic-deadening foods. I substitute Pasta Not! for pasta under my turkey meatballs with sauce. And you can have plenty of Pasta Not! because it's practically calorie-free. If you're craving a big bowl of buttery noodles, trick yourself by eating yellow squash with your favorite seasoning. Never butter unless you want to gain weight. The more Pasta Not! you eat, the leaner you'll be.

3 large yellow squash, peeled
2 large carrots
2 to 3 teaspoons minced or chopped garlic
    (store-bought is fine)
juice from 1/2 lime or store-bought lime juice (optional)

3 large zucchini, peeled
2 tablespoons fat-free chicken stock
1/4 teaspoon black pepper
1/2 teaspoon No-Salt (optional)

Cut or slice squash, carrots and zucchini into thin ribbons with a mandolin slicer or as we Italians do it by hand with a knife with skill.

In a large skillet, heat chicken stock over medium heat. Add garlic and cook for 2 minutes, adding more stock or water if it dries out to quickly.

Add carrot ribbons. Toss in zucchini and squash ribbons, salt and pepper. Cook for 5 to 10 minutes. Keep an eye on it because it is fat-free and may cook quickly and/or dry out.

ROASTED ASPARAGUS BUNDLES

Minutes to Prepare: 5 ◆ Minutes to Cook: 25 ◆ Number of Servings: 4

Asparagus, full of vitamins K, A, and C as well as iron, thiamin, folate, and fiber, is a good choice for when you need an easy go-to vegetable—or when you want to feel less bloated. Did you know that asparagus is a natural diuretic? Fitness pros and models eat asparagus the day before a shoot to help rid the body of excess water. I love to eat these bundles with fish or on top of a salad. And they're great cold the next day as a finger food when I need to munch. Serve it with any lean protein. I love this with fish or on top of your salad.

1 Lb. fresh asparagus spears, tough ends trimmed and discarded (about 5 to 6 stalks per serving)
1/2 teaspoon NoSalt
olive oil cooking spray or 1 tablespoon or less of extra-virgin olive oil

Preheat oven to 400 degrees.

Place asparagus on a baking sheet. Spray with olive oil cooking spray or drizzle with olive oil and sprinkle with NoSalt. Roast 25 to 30 minutes, until tender.

Wrap individual portions of asparagus with asparagus to tie into bundles.

LISA LYNN'S HEALTH-BOOSTING CARROT OVEN FRIES

Minutes to Prepare: 5 ◆ Minutes to Cook: 25 ◆ Number of Servings: 4 to 6

This is my secret way of getting kids who visit my house to eat their veggies. And guess what I have learned in the 25 years of helping people lose weight? That there are lots of grownups who hate veggies too. While the Hidden Valley Ranch seasoning isn't perfect, it does give added flavor and serves as a little motivation to do the right thing: eat vegetables. These carrots are simple to make and inexpensive, which is a good thing because you will never have any leftovers. These go great with turkey or tuna burgers to keep the meal healthy and balanced but still fun.

1 Lb. carrots (about 5 or 6 large, peeled and cut in 4x1/4-inch sticks) or a bag of baby carrots
1 packet Hidden Valley Original Ranch Dressing & Seasoning mix
vegetable cooking spray

Preheat oven to 400.

In a large bowl, combine carrots with olive oil and 1/2 the packet of the Dry Hidden Valley Original Ranch Salad Dressing Seasoning Mix. Toss until well coated.

Spray pan generously with cooking spray. Arrange carrots in single layer on pan and bake 25 to 30 minutes or until crispy.

AUNT HEDWIG'S CABBAGE AND ONIONS TO DIE FOR

Minutes to Prepare: 10 ✦ Minutes to Cook: 20 to 30 ✦ Number of Servings: 6 to 8

Who knew a simple cabbage recipe could be so delicious? Cabbage is a nutritional powerhouse but what most people don't know is that you practically burn more calories eating this vegetable than digesting. It is a great Thermogenic food that revs up your metabolism. My Polish Aunt Hedwig made this recipe and no matter the age, everyone in the family licked their plates clean. We all (even the kids) licked the plate clean. My Grandpa Vinnie liked to add a can of crushed tomatoes to the cabbage while cooking. And would often do so while my Aunt Hedwig left the cabbage unattended for a moment. Feel free to get creative by adding turkey or chicken—add what your family likes. This dish also makes a mellow warming side dish for cold weather roasts. And it may say serves 6 to 8, but if you eat like me it's a serving for one.

1 tablespoon of your favorite vinegar such as cider, white wine, or sherry
2 to 3 tablespoon fat-free chicken broth
sea salt or Himalayan salt and freshly ground black pepper to taste
1 clove garlic minced (optional)

2 medium onions
1 large head of cabbage (I like Savoy best)
1 teaspoon olive oil
1 teaspoon caraway, cumin, fenugreek, or fennel (optional)
1 can crushed tomatoes (optional)

Quarter the cabbage and cut out the core. Slice the cabbage as thinly as possible and set it aside. (You can use a food processor or kitchen mandolin, if you like or cut it by hand.)

Halve, peel, and slice the onions as thinly as possible.

Heat a large pot or deep sauté pan over medium-high heat. Add the oil and chicken broth. When hot, add the onions, sprinkling them with salt, and cook until the onions wilt, about 3 minutes. Add the cabbage and garlic (if using), sprinkling with salt again and stir to combine.

Reduce heat to low, and cook, covered, until the vegetables are extremely tender, about 30 minutes, stirring occasionally. If using, add caraway, cumin, fenugreek, or fennel at this point. Add crushed tomatoes as well if using; this turns it into a yummy cabbage stew

Add a tablespoon or two of water to keep vegetables from sticking if necessary.

MUSHROOMS AND SPINACH ITALIAN-STYLE

Minutes to Prepare: 10 ◆ Minutes to Cook: 10 ◆ Number of Servings: 4

We may joke about spinach making us strong thanks to the old Popeye cartoons, but the truth is, spinach really is a nutritional powerhouse and great metabolic booster. Eat as much of this as you want. Try it cold as a salad too. You can add shredded chicken or shrimp or add more water or broth to make a great slimming soup.

4 tablespoon fat-free chicken broth
1 small onion, chopped
14 oz. fresh mushrooms (I adore baby bellas)
10 oz. clean fresh spinach, (chop if desired)
Salt and Pepper to taste

olive oil spray
2 cloves of garlic, chopped (or 2 tablespoons store-bought minced garlic)
1 tablespoon balsamic vinegar

Spray Skillet and heat fat-free chicken broth in a large skillet over medium-high heat. Sauté onion and garlic until they start to become tender.

Add mushrooms and sauté until they begin to shrink, about 3 to 4 minutes.

Toss in the spinach stirring constantly for a few minutes or until spinach is wilted.

Add the balsamic vinegar, reduce heat to low, and simmer until the liquid is almost completely absorbed. Season with salt and pepper to taste.

FAT-MELTING ONIONS AND PEPPER

Minutes to Prepare: 10 ◆ Minutes to Cook: 10 ◆ Number of Servings: 4

Everyone needs to know how to make killer onions and peppers. My Aunt Angie showed me this version and yummy-lean. These veggies not only turn up the dial on your metabolism but they are delicious hot or cold. I love the smell permeating the house when I'm preparing this dish and I adore it when my kids walk in and go "Yummm! What's for dinner?" and start grabbing at these veggies. I love to top my chicken breast or white fish with these colorful veggies. Make extra and toss them into your salads and soups. Onions and peppers should be a staple at every barbecue—with turkey or salmon sausage, of course.

1 medium-sized red pepper (use frozen or sliced vegetables from your supermarket's salad bar if short on time)
1 medium yellow onion
olive oil spray
salt and pepper (optional)

1 medium-sized yellow pepper
1 medium-sized green pepper
1 medium-sized orange pepper
2 cloves garlic (optional)
2 tablespoons red wine vinegar

Start chopping. Cut your onions in half then quarters. Chop the onions in such a way that you end up with half circle strips. Slice peppers into long strips about 1/8 of an inch thick.

Chop garlic into smallest mince possible.

Spray medium skillet with olive oil spray and heat on medium. Be sure spray covers every part of the pan.

Throw your sliced onions and peppers* into the skillet and cook for 10 minutes, stirring occasionally. Turn heat down after 10 minutes to low to keep onions from burning and to allow them to soften. Add garlic at the end when you turn down the heat. Want more spice? Add a pinch of salt and pepper for flavor.

Pour 2 tablespoons of red wine vinegar into the skillet and you're ready to eat.

*Roasting is easy too. Simply place your peppers on a foil-lined and lightly olive-oil sprayed sheet pan for 40 minutes until they are completely winkled and charred. Turn them twice while roasting. Remove from pan and immediately cover with foil and set aside for 30 minutes or until peppers are cool enough to handle. Remove stem from each pepper and cut into quarters. Remove seeds and place peppers in a bowl along with any juices. Cover with plastic and refrigerate for up to two weeks.

ZUCCHINI-INTO-YOUR-BIKINI PARMESAN CRISPS

Minutes to Prepare: 15 ◆ Minutes to Cook: 30 ◆ Number of Servings: 4

This is how you break the potato chip habit. Why grab crispy chips and blow your diet when you can eat these? I make these at least once a week. What makes this recipes extra lean? No egg yolk and very, very little oil. Put some sauce on these and you have a fast and easy pizza that won't stop your weight loss.

2 medium zucchini (about 1 pound total) (approximately 1/4 cup Italian bread crumbs cooking spray

1/4 cup freshly grated Parmesan cheese 3/4 ounce)

Preheat the oven to 450 degrees. Coat baking sheet with cooking spray. (You can also cook these in a toaster oven where they heat up fast and get crispier even faster)

Slice zucchini into 1/4 inch thick rounds. In a medium bowl spray with spray oil and toss the zucchini to cover.

In a small bowl combine the Parmesan, bread crumbs. Dip each round into the Parmesan mixture, coating it evenly on both sides, pressing the coating on to stick, and place in a single layer on the prepared baking sheet.

Bake the zucchini rounds until browned and crisp, 25 to 30 minutes. Remove with spatula. Serve immediately.

PORTOBELLO UN-PIZZA

Minutes to Prepare: 5 ◆ Minutes to Cook: 12 ◆ Number of Servings: 1

When I was little I was a chubette. Here's an embarrassing confession: All my relatives used to call me Lisa Pizza—and I didn't get that name for nothin'. I craved pizza and could never get enough. My pizza craving didn't go away as I grew older, either. I could never stop at one slice and then I could never work off in the gym. I finally found a lean solution: While my family eats pizza, I eat Portobello UN-Pizza guilt-free. Get creative. You'll never miss the cheese if you add shrimp or turkey meatballs, and your flatter stomach will show up sooner. Make it Thermogenic by adding 3 ounces of precooked chicken breast. These pizzas can also be made on squash slices for an even lighter meal that fills you up, not out. And guess what? My family now fights over these.

1 Portobello mushroom, 4 to 5 inches in diameter
3 tablespoons marinara or other tomato-based sauce
(look for no sugar added and low-fat)

olive oil spray
NoSalt and black pepper to taste
1 teaspoon reduced-fat Parmesan, grated
(optional)

Preheat oven to 425. If mushroom has a stem, slice it off close to the cap (reserve for soups or sauces). Spray cap with olive oil and place stem side up on a rimmed baking sheet or pan. Sprinkle lightly with NoSalt and pepper. Bake 15 minutes until mushrooms are hot. Spread sauce on cap and top with cheese if using.

KALE CHIPS

Minutes to Prepare: 5 ◆ Minutes to Cook: 30 ◆ Number of Servings: Why measure?

Kale is big on the health food radar these days. Truth is, I don't love Kale, but I do love to munch and crunch during anxious times so this is just what I need. An awesome client who has lots 60 pounds turned me onto this recipe. A great potato chip replacement and it's so easy your kids can make these. If you want to cut down on the oil, use a spray—you won't have to use a bag then either. Be creative and use your favorite spices. And try substituting with string beans or whatever veggies you have in the house. Just remember to adjust cooking time.

big bunch of kale greens
1 teaspoon balsamic vinegar
salt-free Mrs. Dash (optional)

1 tablespoon olive oil
sea salt
large zip-top bag

Wash kale greens and dry thoroughly with paper towels. Tear off 2-inch portions of the leaves. Discard stems as they are bitter. Place the leaves in zip-top bag. Add olive oil and balsamic vinegar. Close bag and "massage" to distribute evenly. (The bag keeps fingers from getting messy)

Remove leaves and place in single layer onto cookie sheet lined with parchment paper. Sprinkle with sea salt or Mrs. Dash if using.

Roast in 350-degree oven for 30 minutes.

THE INCREDIBLE METABOLIC-BOOSTING EGG WHITE

If you're trying to boost your metabolism so you can finally lose weight and you hate fish, egg whites (right after the Complete Protein Shake) are your new best friend. They are one of the best sources of protein and have no fat. Not just for breakfast anymore, egg whites make one of the best quick delicious meals. Armed with these delicious and filling recipes you will never have an excuse to not eat lean and clean. And don't forget about the basic hard-boiled egg—just discard the yolk. Did you know that one yolk has 7 grams of fat? That's almost half of your daily fat allowance of 15 to 20 grams when trying to lose weight. And don't buy into the ads claiming that yolks contain "good" fat. If you're out to lose weight, you have to reduce your fat intake, no and's, if's, or but's. Keep a stash of hard-boiled egg whites in your refrigerator for those moments when you need to pop something into your mouth.

Egg whites don't have any fat so they cook much faster than yolked eggs—so keep your eye on them. If you want fluffier, fuller eggs buy them fresh and whip them to get air into them. Want more? Add a little water or even seltzer—the bubbles add even more air. Need more flavor? Add more spices, not fats like oils or cheeses. And skip the mayo, make egg white salad using mustard or salsa. Don't feel like messing around with a recipe? Simply add 1 tablespoon of salsa to 3 egg whites ad make the Salsa Scramble.

POMODORINI CON UOVE DI FABRIZIO

Minutes to Prepare: 5 ♦ Minutes to Cook: 10 ♦ Number of Servings: 2

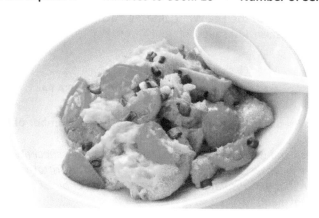

My Grandfather used to make this dish for me with his ciambotto. It makes egg whites seem like a special treat.

1 medium onion sliced
chopped parsley (optional)

1/2 can crushed, peeled tomatoes
olive or canola oil spray

8 egg whites   salt and pepper (optional)

Spray a small fry pan with olive or canola oil spray and sauté onions until wilted and soft. Add a little water if too dry. Add tomatoes and parsley (if using) and cook for 5 to 10 minutes stirring often.

As tomatoes simmer, gently break 8 eggs separating the white and discarding the yolk. Poach whites in boiling water until cooked to your liking. Add a salad on the side or any left-over vegetables directly to the eggs and you've got metabolism-boosting meal that's done in 10 minutes and delicious.

EGG WHITE BITES

Minutes to Prepare: 10   ◆   Minutes to Cook: 6 to 8   ◆   Number of Servings: 6

I always have these in my refrigerator; they are great to pop into your mouth when you just gotta munch. Your whole family will love them and be healthier eating these Egg White Bites. They pack great in kids' lunch boxes and in yours too. Top salads with them or have them as a lean snack to help reach your protein quota. My son Kyle loves to make these and that gets him to eat them too. Mothers of wrestlers: This will get a big smile as it will help your son stay healthy and make his weight class. Egg White Bites make a great post-workout snack, refueling your muscles.

2 cups Egg Beater egg whites or 12 egg whites   cooking spray
2 plum tomatoes, chopped, seeded, and drained   1 teaspoon chopped basil (optional)
1 teaspoon chopped garlic (optional)   NoSalt and pepper to taste

Preheat oven to 350 degrees. Spray a nonstick muffin tin with cooking spray. Drop one egg white into each well of the muffin tin. Place 1 tsp chopped tomato on each egg white and sprinkle with NoSalt and pepper, if desired.

Place on center rack of oven and bake for 6-8 minutes or until egg whites reach desired doneness.

Get creative. Add any vegetable to the Egg White Bite. Spinach, asparagus, broccoli, peppers and onions, an oriental blend—all are great. Add salsa, hot sauce, or your favorite spice.

SALMON AND ASPARAGUS FRITTATA

Minutes to Prepare: 10   ◆   Minutes to Cook: 20   ◆   Number of Servings: 4

My husband doesn't cook much and when he does it's a treat. This is Jeff's specialty. We all look forward to Sunday brunch and hope there will be leftovers for lunch on Monday. This frittata makes an awesome dinner or lunch, too. For a salmon touch that will absolutely dazzle you, try Vital Choice's salmon bacon (vitalchoice.com). It's perfect for that extra special meal.

12 egg whites (lightly beaten)   salt and pepper (optional)
olive oil spray   1 cup chopped onion
1/2 cup red bell pepper, diced   8 oz. salmon fillet, skin removed and cut into
1/2 teaspoon oregano   bite-sized pieces

Preheat broiler. Combine egg whites with salt and pepper (if using) in a bowl.

Spray 12-inch oven-proof skillet over medium high-heat and cook onion, bell pepper, and oregano, stirring occasionally until vegetables are somewhat soft, about 3 minutes.

Add asparagus and cook 3 minutes. Add salmon and cook until opaque, approximately 3 minutes.

Pour egg mixture into skillet and reduce heat to low, stirring occasionally until eggs begin to set but are still wet on top, about 5 minutes. Cook for an additional 5 minutes without stirring. Transfer skillet to broiler and broil until golden 2 to 3 minutes. Serve with salad.

THE HEARTY (I'M STARVING!) OMELET

Minutes to Prepare: None ◆ Minutes to Cook: 5 ◆ Number of Servings: 2

At my house, this is the I'm-starving-I-could-eat-a-horse omelet. In those moments, we get very creative; I open the fridge and take out whatever I have available (usually ciambotta) and scramble it in a pan with three egg whites per person. Add a sprinkle of Parmesan cheese and you have a meal fast. Make one day a week omelet night to help you lose weight faster. You can mix in any food on the metabolic boosting food lists starting on page 89. Just remember, if you don't see a food listed, don't eat it. If I don't list a food that means it's not good for weight loss. Old food faves like bacon, cheese (even low fat) and any kind of red meat do not boost your metabolism.

6 egg whites   spray oil
your favorite leftover or ingredient

Spray pan. Add 3 whisked egg whites. Fry until solid. Add filling, flip omelet half over to close. Cook additional 1 to 2 minutes. Serve. Repeat with additional egg whites.

EGG WHITE FLORENTINE IN A TOMATO CUP

Minutes to Prepare: 5 ◆ Minutes to Cook: 25 ◆ Number of Servings: 4

This is the perfect combination of flavors and textures, which is important when eating clean. We eat with all of our senses and that's why it's critical to get creative if you're going to live lean. It's not just good for your metabolism, it also keeps you from getting bored.

8 large egg whites (separated) at room temperature
    and already whipped
olive oil spray or 1 teaspoon olive oil
1 10 oz. package frozen spinach, thawed and
    squeezed of all excess liquid

4 large beefsteak tomatoes
1/4 cup minced shallots
1/4 cup low sodium chicken broth
1/4 cup grated Parmesan cheese
salt & pepper (optional)

Preheat oven to 400 degrees. Slice off top of each tomato and using a melon baller, scoop out the insides of the tomatoes, do not discard. Make sure to leave the outside intact to form a cup. Place the hollowed out tomatoes on a foil lined baking sheet.

Heat a medium nonstick skillet over medium heat (already sprayed with oil spray). Add shallots and cook for 2 minutes or until translucent.

Whisk in broth and cook for 2 to 3 minutes or until warm. Add spinach and tomato pulp and cook, stirring 2 to 3 minutes or until liquid is evaporated. Stir in 1/2 the Parmesan cheese and salt and pepper if desired (cheese has enough salt trust me)

Fill one tomato with 1/3 cup of spinach. Then form a small well in the center. Carefully pour egg whites into center of the spinach well; repeat with remaining tomatoes.

Sprinkle each tomato with remaining Parmesan cheese and cook for 15 to 20 minutes or until egg whites are set. Serve immediately.

Rushed? Cook the tomatoes while cooking egg whites spinach together. Then put the warm mixture into the heated tomato shells. This cuts the time in half.

THE SALAD OMELET

Minutes to Prepare: 10 ◆ Minutes to Cook: 5 ◆ Number of Servings: 2

1/2 cup grape tomatoes
1 teaspoon extra virgin olive oil or olive oil spray
salt and pepper to taste (optional)
3 cups mixed baby greens or mescalin mix
  (my preference)

6 large egg whites or 1 1/2 cups egg-white substitute
1/4 cup roughly chopped flat leaf parsley
1 tablespoon red wine vinegar

Position a rack on the shelf closest to broiler and preheat broiler on high.

Toss the tomatoes with the vinegar and spray with olive oil or use 1/2 the teaspoon. Season with salt and pepper: set aside

Warm a medium nonstick oven-ready skillet over medium-low heat. Whisk the egg whites in a large bowl until foamy and doubled in volume. Season with salt and pepper and whisk in parsley. Add the remaining olive oil to the skillet or better yet spray it.

Pour egg whites into the skillet and swirl to cover entire skillet. Cook, without stirring, until the whites are almost set and light brown on the bottom, about 3 minutes.

Transfer the skillet under the broiler and cook until the omelet sets and begins to brown, about 30 seconds. Spoon half the tomato salad onto half the omelet and fold the omelet over filling. Transfer omelet to a serving platter and arrange the remaining tomato salad on top. Serve with baby greens on side or you can stuff the omelet with the baby greens—that's my favorite.

COFFEE CUP SCRAMBLE
(THE THREE-MINUTE EGG WHITE)

Minutes to Prepare: 1 ◆ **Minutes to Cook: 20** ◆ **Number of Servings: 1**

This recipe works for those hard-to-get-protein times like vacations, when at the office, or when you're going to have an extremely long day and need warm real food. I like this recipe because my kids and husband will eat them. Breakfast is the most important meal of the day, but that doesn't mean you default to eating carbohydrates. Protein provides sustainable energy and keeps our minds sharp and our bodies ready to go. When you need a quick protein pick-me-up, try this one. You can add turkey sausage, vegetables, salmon, or your favorite spice and make it your own.

2 to 3 egg whites or equivalent amount of
    egg white substitute

1 teaspoon mild salsa
spray oil

Spray to coat a 12 to 16 oz. microwave-safe coffee mug with cooking spray. Add egg whites and beat in salsa until blended.

Microwave on high 45 seconds and stir and microwave an additional 30 to 45 seconds or until cooked. Microwave cooking times may vary so adjust accordingly.

SLIMMING SOUPS

Soup is one of the best kept secrets when it comes to losing weight. It's fast filling and if it's packed with the right ingredients like light broths (fat-free and low-sodium of course), vegetables, and lean proteins, it's good for your metabolism. These recipes are simple to make and so delicious you'll crave them day after day. These soups have minimal calories and are full of thermogenic vegetables that will rev up your metabolism. Soups will not only keep you feeling full but they will help you lose weight faster and they are a great way to keep you hydrated. Finally, a comfort food that's good for you.

Soup is one of my favorites no matter what the season. Remember: It's your soup, so you can enjoy them hot or cold and add the thermogenic condiments according to your taste. Like it thick? Simply puree any of these soups for a thicker consistency. (Use caution when pureeing hot liquids.) Soup is a great way to keep you full and melt fat off your belly.

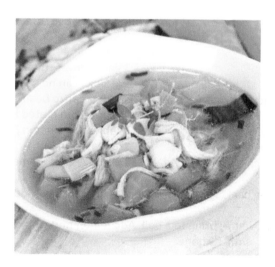

CHICKEN SOUP FOR THE METABOLISM

Minutes to Prepare: 15 ◆ Minutes to Cook: 30 ◆ Number of Servings: 4

There is nothing like good, Old-Fashioned Chicken Soup. It's a classic American comfort food. Flavorful stock, fresh-cooked chicken and fresh vegetables (minus the diet-sabotaging egg noodles) make this the ultimate comfort food that won't hurt your metabolism while hitting the spot.

8 cups chicken stock or fat-free, lower-sodium
    chicken broth
2 cups diagonally sliced carrot

2 (4 oz.) skinless, bone-in chicken thighs
1 (12 oz.) skinless, bone-in chicken breast half
2 cups diagonally sliced celery

1 cup chopped onion

1/2 teaspoon black pepper

1/2 teaspoon kosher salt

Celery leaves (optional)

Combine the first three ingredients in a large pot over medium-high heat; bring to a boil. Reduce heat and simmer 20 minutes.

Remove chicken from pan; let stand for 10 minutes. Remove chicken from bones; shred meat into bite-sized pieces. Discard bones.

Add carrot, celery, and onion to pan; cover and simmer for 10 minutes. Add chicken, salt, and black pepper; cook until done. Garnish with celery leaves, if desired.

LEMONY SPINACH SOUP

Minutes to Prepare: 15 ◆ Minutes to Cook: 30 ◆ Number of Servings: 4

This is one of the most light and refreshing soups you'll ever try. This soup can be turned into a meal by adding strips of chicken or shrimp. For a vegetarian version of this lemony soup, use organic or lower-sodium vegetable broth in place of chicken broth.

1 teaspoon extra-virgin olive oil

2 thinly sliced green onions

4 cups fat-free, lower-sodium chicken broth

2 cups water

1 tablespoon chopped fresh oregano

1/2 teaspoon freshly ground black pepper

1 (6 oz.) package fresh baby spinach

3 garlic cloves, thinly sliced

1 (15 oz.) can no-salt-added chickpeas
(garbanzo beans), drained

1 tablespoon grated lemon rind

1 tablespoon lemon juice

1/8 teaspoon salt

1/3 cup grated Parmesan cheese (optional)

Heat a large saucepan over high heat. Add olive oil and swirl to coat. Add garlic and onions and sauté 30 seconds, stirring constantly.

Add chicken broth and 2 cups water; bring to a boil. Add lemon rind, and chickpeas.

Cover and cook 10 minutes or until it's done.

Stir in oregano and next four ingredients (through spinach). Ladle 1 3/4 cups soup into each of 4 bowls. Top each serving with about sprinkle of parmesan cheese.

GIGI'S ZUPPA DI SCAROLA
(ESCAROLE SOUP)

Minutes to Prepare: 15 ◆ Minutes to Cook: 30 ◆ Number of Servings: 4

Growing up, my younger brother Gary ("Gigi") was the cook in our house, and one of the things he made very well was escarole soup. It was probably the only healthy thing we ate. It is one of the easiest, most delicious soups to make. This version is a metabolic-boosting version so the carbohydrates and fat are removed. This soup can easily be made into a meal by adding thin strips of chicken pulled of the bone or floating some shrimp in it.

On a weekend as a special treat I'll add turkey sausage.

1 head escarole (cut into bite-sized pieces)
4 cups fat-free, low-sodium chicken broth
salt/ pepper

2 tablespoon carrots, chopped
2 cups water
Parmesan cheese, optional

Simmer escarole, carrots, and chicken broth seasoned with salt for 20 minutes. Add black pepper and water, stir well. Ladle hot soup into bowls. Sprinkle with Parmesan cheese if desired.

ZUPPA DI SPOSALIZIO
(ITALIAN WEDDING SOUP GONE LEAN)

Minutes to Prepare: 10 ◆ Minutes to Cook: 15 ◆ Number of Servings: 4

If you grew up Italian, you know we never waste one single meatball. We eat them every possible way. And since the turkey meatballs in this book are so lean, you can eat them every day. This is a very simple and fast soup you can make in 20 minutes or less and leave the table feeling satisfied without slowing your metabolism.

4 cups fat free chicken broth
2 tsp iodized salt (optional)
4 cups of romaine lettuce leaves (spinach or
    escarole work well)

1 small onion-sliced into rings
2 cups of water
turkey meatballs (from recipe on page 203)

Put broth and onion in a large pot and cook over medium heat for 3 to 5 minutes until hot. Add turkey meatballs and cook 2 to 3 more minutes or until warm. Do not boil or overcook. Add romaine leaves at the end as they cook very fast. Ladle into large soup bowl and mangia! Want seconds? Go for it.

GET LEAN GAZPACHO

Minutes to Prepare: 15 ◆ Minutes to Cook: N/A ◆ Number of Servings: 4

Gazpacho is one of the easiest soups to make and it's one of the healthiest. It's also super delicious. This recipe is leaner and cleaner because I don't add oil which jacks up the calories. I also like my gazpacho chunkier so I make it in a food processor by pulsing it until the desired thickness is reached. No food processor? No problem, use your blender. My favorite addition for a no-cook meal that absolutely rocks your socks off and doesn't slow your metabolism: Add crab meat or shrimp.

2 roma (plum) tomatoes, chopped
1/2 green bell pepper, chopped
1/2 small red onion, chopped
2 cups tomato juice
1/2 teaspoon dried oregano

1/2 cucumber, chopped
1/2 red bell pepper, chopped
1 clove garlic, minced
2 teaspoon beef bouillon granules
1/2 teaspoon dried basil

1/4 teaspoon celery salt
1/8 teaspoon ground black pepper
1 1/2 teaspoon red wine vinegar

1/4 teaspoon salt
1 1/2 teaspoon Worcestershire sauce

Puree roma tomatoes, cucumber, green and red bell peppers, red onion, and garlic in food processor or blender about 30 seconds. Add tomato juice, beef bouillon granules, oregano, basil, celery salt, salt, black pepper, Worcestershire sauce, and red wine vinegar. Pulse a few times to mix. Pour into a bowl and chill at least 1 hour.

Like your gazpacho thicker? Pulse tomatoes in the food processor until desired texture is achieved. Pour into a bowl. Repeat with the bell peppers (I use red, green, and yellow) and onions, and pour into bowl. Repeat again with cucumbers. This allows you to control the texture of all the vegetables. Finally, add the bouillon, fresh oregano, fresh basil, seasonings, Worcestershire, and red wine vinegar and pulse to mix. Add to bowl with the other processed veggies. In a rush? Use frozen peppers or precut ones form your market salad bar.

ROMAN EGG DROP SOUP
(EGG WHITE DROP THE POUNDS SOUP)

Minutes to Prepare: 5 ◆ Minutes to Cook: 5 ◆ Number of Servings: 2 to 3

Egg drop soup is very popular in Rome, but it is so high in cholesterol. I make a leaner version that is good for boosting your metabolism rather than slowing it down. You'll never miss the yolks—and that's where all the fat is. Removing the yolk saves you 7 grams of fat per yolk. If you were to add 2 eggs you would have used up almost all of your 20 grams of fat per day budget. However using only the white of the egg is great for tightening and firming your skin, including the skin on your face. This is why body builders and fitness models eat egg whites all of the time. This is a fast, delicious, and very satisfying soup that you can make in 2 minutes. You can add more vegetables or have a huge salad along with it.

4 cups chicken broth
1 tablespoon chopped scallions

6 egg whites
Add your favorite vegetables (optional)

Place broth in medium size pot and bring to slow boil. Whip/beat egg whites until thick. Gently and slowly pour egg whites into simmering broth stirring gently. Continue to stir, simmer for 2-3 minutes. Serve Topped scallions.

Need more flavor? Add 1/2 cup of sweet onions. Simple sauté them in pan before adding broth for 1 to 2 minutes.

MELT FAT MINESTRONE
(ITALIAN CABBAGE SOUP)

Minutes to Prepare: 15 ◆ Minutes to Cook: 40 ◆ Number of Servings: 8

If you think cabbage soup is effective when it comes to weight loss, wait until you try this. The difference? You'll actually like this one. This soup is one of the staples in my house. I leave out the pasta and add it to my husband's and the kids' soup bowl since they need the carbs and I don't. I love it for a healthy weeknight recipe because it's loaded with vegetables and everyone loves it. Have gluten-sensitive kids? Use rice for them instead of pasta. I make this my meal by adding some scrod, halibut, or shrimp. Add a salad and you're so full you won't be looking for dessert. Remember veggies are free and so is the broth as it's so clean. So use as much as you want.

Spray olive oil
1/4 head of cabbage, shredded*
1/4 pound of green beans, cut into 1 inch pieces
2 cups of fat free beef broth (vegetable soups work
    for vegans, too)
9 cups of water
3 small zucchini chopped

1 garlic clove, chopped
3 stalks of celery, diced
3 carrots sliced
1 small can of tomato paste
1 Small can of kidney beans
1 cup of onions

Spray pan with olive oil spray and sauté onions, garlic, parsley, celery, cabbage, carrots, and green beans until wilted.
    Add tomato paste, beef broth, and water and simmer for 20 minutes or until cooked.
    Add beans and zucchini and cook for 5 to 20 more minutes.
    Serve topped with a dash of parmesan cheese.

*Not a cabbage eater? Substitute your favorite vegetable like yellow squash or spinach. Need more flavor? Add dash of hot sauce or sprinkle in your favorite seasoning, like McCargo's Signature Blend or Mrs. Dash.

VERY QUICK VEGETARIAN CHILI

Minutes to Prepare: 10 ◆ Minutes to Cook: 25 ◆ Number of Servings: 6

Finally, comfort food that is good for you. This is a great way to reduce calories after a not-so-good eating day. This recipe is practically free it's so healthy. Need protein? Add some cooked turkey chunks instead of beans to keep calories low. And when you're pressed for time, you can always use low-sodium taco seasoning (aka Turkey Joes in my house) and add loads of veggies. I like to add green vegetables and use "steamer" frozen veggies so I don't have to spend my time chopping. Be sure to make extra and freeze it in single storage containers so it's always ready to grab and go. Enjoy.

2 teaspoons canola oil
1 cup chopped red bell pepper
1 teaspoon ground cumin
3 cloves of garlic, minced

1 cup chopped onion
2 teaspoon chili powder
1 teaspoon dried oregano
1 (4.5 oz.) can chopped green chilies

1/4 cup water
1 (14.5 oz.) can no-salt-added, diced tomatoes,
     undrained
Precooked turkey pieces

1 (15 oz.) can black beans, drained
1 can (14 oz.) low-sodium, vegetable broth
3 tablespoon chopped fresh cilantro
6 lime wedges

Heat the oil in a pan on medium-high heat. Add the onion and bell pepper; sauté until soft (about 3 to 5 minutes).

Add chili powder, cumin, oregano, garlic and green chilies. Cook 1 minute. Stir in water, black beans, diced tomatoes and vegetable broth. Bring to a boil; cover; reduce heat and simmer 15-20 minutes. Stir in cilantro.

Serve with limes wedges.

SALADS

Salads are not just for the salad bowl. These awesome, slimming, thermogenic wonders can be sautéed if you crave warm comfort food. They work great under your favorite protein—place your favorite fish or chicken on top of a salad instead of pasta. Salads are especially great as fillers, stopping you from overindulging on a perhaps-not-so-fat-free main course. Anytime you want to fill up, try adding some fat-free chicken broth or your favorite bouillon over you salad for a delicious, hot, almost-calorie-free soup. The recipes that follow are based on the most popular salads we eat in the United States, but they've been made over to boost your metabolism.

LISA'S FAMOUS SAUTÉED SALAD

Minutes to Prepare: 5 ◆ Minutes to Cook: 10 ◆ Number of Servings: 2

This is one of my all-time go-to food favorites. Sometimes I'm just not in the mood for another cold salad and, frankly, I just don't find them very filling. But throw a boring salad into a pan and toss it around until it's lightly cooked—delicious. I'll make a meal out of it by adding some shrimp, scallops, or shredded chicken breast. It makes a great filling to wrap a fish fillet around. And I love to throw in a cup of cooked broccoli. Add water or fat-free broth and you have instant slimming soup. Best of all? Romaine lettuce (which should be a staple you always have on hand) has almost no calories. So if you're hungry—make more.

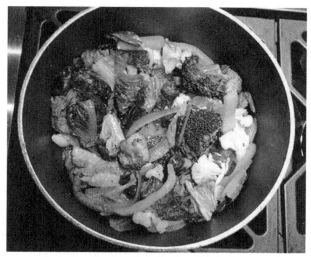

spray olive oil or 1/2 tablespoon or less extra virgin olive oil (use as little as possible)
1 small, sweet onion such as white or Vidalia, thinly sliced
3 heads Romaine lettuce (substitute chopped escarole or broccoli rabe if you wish)

1/4 teaspoon NoSalt
grated Parmesan (optional)

Heat oil in 12-inch skillet over medium heat. Add onion and cook, stirring often, for 10 minutes or until golden. Lower heat if onion is browning too quickly; don't let it brown.

Add Romaine to skillet and cook, turning occasionally, for about 2 to 3 minutes, until leaves are tender yet still crunchy. Sprinkle with salt substitute. Garnish with grated cheese, if desired.

CLEANEST SKINNY CAESAR SALAD

Minutes to Prepare: 10 to 15 ◆ Number of Servings: 2

Caesar salad is my go-to food when it comes to "What should I eat?" when I'm trying to keep it clean. Caesar salads make eating healthier easy—as long as you have the right recipe. You'll never feel deprived again once you try this light, lean Caesar salad. You'll save loads of calories and money because this salad is better than anything you'll find eating out. My friends tell me they think it's better than "the real fattening version".

1 large garlic clove, chopped
Juice of 1/2 lemon
1 teaspoon Worcestershire
Croutons (optional)
Parmesan
4 cups chopped romaine

2 teaspoons Dijon mustard
1/4 cup fat-free chicken broth or extra-virgin olive oil
4 anchovies, rinsed
Grilled chicken or shrimp*
Salt and pepper

Combine Worcestershire, Dijon, anchovies, lemon, and garlic in blender, slowly adding the chicken broth or extra virgin olive oil.

Mix with the chopped romaine and top with grilled chicken or shrimp and Parmesan cheese. Generously season with salt and pepper.

*I marinate the chicken in nonfat Italian dressing.

LISA'S BE-HEALTHY SALAD

Minutes to Prepare: 10 to 15 ◆ Number of Servings: 4

This is the most important "Health Recipe" I will ever give you. If you want to lose weight and be healthy, you need to eat 10 veggies every day. The vitamins, minerals, and fiber in my Be-Healthy Salad keep you healthy and feeling full while satisfying the urge to crunch. This salad helps you get them all in and can be heated if you don't feel like another cold salad. It's a meal on its own, but you can also add chicken, turkey, boiled egg whites, chunk light tuna (packed in water), shrimp or fish. Serve it as a side salad. The dressing can be made ahead of time and stored in the refrigerator. Double up on the ingredients so you have a salad ready to go for lunch tomorrow.

SIMPLE SALAD DRESSING

1 to 2 teaspoons red wine vinegar
1 1/2 tablespoon fresh lemon juice
dash NoSalt

canola oil cooking spray
1/4 teaspoon freshly ground black pepper (optional)

Combine ingredients, stirring with whisk. Cover and chill.

SALAD

3 cups romaine lettuce, chopped (or any lettuce)
1/4 cup red onion, sliced vertically
1/2 tomato, sliced
1/4 red pepper
1/4 cup carrots, peeled and sliced
1 tablespoon Fiber One cereal (optional)

1/4 cucumber, thinly sliced
1/4 cup radishes, thinly sliced
1/4 yellow pepper
1/4 cup purple cabbage
1/4 cup broccoli florets

Place chopped lettuce in a large bowl; add rest of vegetables and toss to combine.

Sprinkle with Fiber One cereal for texture, if desired.

Pour dressing over salad, tossing gently to coat or dress with your favorite store-bought salad dressing (go fat-free). My favorite is Ken's Raspberry Walnut Vinaigrette. Store-bought brands are not necessarily perfectly clean dressings, but they work in a pinch and are a far better option than any fast food you might end up eating.

CRUNCHY CABBAGE SLAW

Minutes to Prepare: 15 ◆ Number of Servings: 10 ◆ Yield: 2/3 cup

This is my family's all-time favorite way to eat their veggies, particularly when we barbecue at the lake. I've never had a complaint about this calcium and vitamin-filled recipe—even from finicky kids. The dressing isn't perfect, but it's a much better choice than eating out. The warm dressing won't wilt the hardy cabbage, but it will make the leaves crisp-tender as they marinate. If you're in a hurry, buy the prepackaged slaw mix in your local market. When salad is done, you can warm the entire dish for a tasty treat. This slaw is fast, easy, and irresistibly delicious. A great side for your chicken breast.

3 cups green cabbage, shredded
1 cup red bell pepper, julienne cut
Walnut
sunflower seeds or 1/3 cup Fiber One cereal (optional)

1 cups red cabbage, shredded
Ken's or Wishbone low-fat or fat-free Raspberry
Vinaigrette (warm it up for a special treat)

Pour dressing over cabbage, bell pepper, and onions in a large bowl; toss well. Sprinkle with salt substitute if desired. Cover and chill 2 hours; stirring occasionally.

Garnish with Fiber One cereal or sunflower seeds before serving.

GREEN APPLE WALDORF SALAD

Minutes to Prepare: 15 ◆ Number of Servings: 4

Eating an apple with or before dinner is one of the oldest tricks in the book when it comes to fighting hunger. Try this with a green apple and you'll be amazed. This is a great salad for those days when you just can't get full. Mayo-free, it is a perfect blend of different flavors and textures to satisfy your sweet tooth. You'll want to make extra so there's some for the next day, just don't dress it until you're ready to eat it.

1/8 cup walnut halves
1/2 cup shredded carrot
6 oz. cooked chicken breast (leftovers are great)
1/2 lemon juiced
2 tablespoons minced flat-leaf parsley for garnish
   (optional)

1 large crisp apple such as Granny Smith or Gala
1 head Boston lettuce, trimmed, washed, and dried
   (or substitute fresh spinach)
1/2 lemon zest, finely grated

If you'd like toasted walnuts (raw is perfectly fine to toss in, too), preheat the oven to 350 degrees F. Spread the nuts on a baking sheets and toast in the oven for 8 to 10 minutes. Cool and break the nuts up into small pieces.

Halve, core and cut the apples into 3/4-inch pieces, leaving skin intact. Add apples and carrots to bowl and sprinkle with the lemon juice; then toss with fat-free raspberry walnut vinaigrette (or try pomegranate vinaigrette). Cover and refrigerate if not serving immediately.

When ready to serve, toss walnuts into the salad. Arrange the lettuce leaves (or spinach) on a large platter or divide them among 4 salad plates. Place the chicken and salad on the lettuce or spinach and serve.

CHINESE CHICKEN SALAD

Minutes to Prepare: 15 ◆ Number of Servings: 4

It's undeniably one of the most popular salads in America but did you know it's also one of the unhealthiest? Most versions of this that you'll find in national restaurant chains are nutritional disasters, bogged down by too much dressing and too many fried noodles. This lighter, cleaner version is true to Wolfgang Puck's original inspiration, but with about a third of the calories.

1 head Napa cabbage
1/2 tablespoon sugar
1/3 cup store-bought Asian vinaigrette
1 cup fresh cilantro leaves
1/4 cup sliced almonds, toasted

1/2 head red cabbage
2 cups chopped or shredded cooked chicken (freshly
   grilled or store-bought rotisserie chicken)
1 cup canned mandarin oranges, drained
Salt and black pepper to taste

Slice cabbages in half lengthwise and remove cores. Then slice cabbage into thin strips. Toss with the sugar in a large bowl.

If the chicken is cold, toss with a few tablespoons of vinaigrette and heat in a microwave at 50% power. Add chicken, cilantro, mandarins, almonds, and remaining vinaigrette to cabbage. Toss to combine. Season with salt and pepper, if desired.

	My Chinese Chicken vs.	A National Restaurant Chain's Version
Calories	380	1,430
Saturated Fat	3.5	16
Carbohydrates	23	93
Cost per Serving	$3.50	$13.99

MIRACLE IN A SALAD

Minutes to Prepare: 15 ◆ Number of Servings: 4 to 6

This is one of the best and most eclectic salads you'll ever eat. When you're in the mood for change but don't feel like breaking your diet, it's good to try something different like this salad with its combination of satisfying spicy and sweet flavors and hunger-curbing appeal. One of the first tricks I learned as a personal trainer was: If you can't get your clients to eat healthier, tell them to eat raspberries because they are fill of fiber. Fiber acts like sponge helping transport fat and cholesterol out of the body. Choose the freshest baby greens you can find; they're higher in nutrients and offer an incredible taste.

1 cup fresh raspberries
1/2 cup snap peas
1/2 large red onion, thinly sliced
1/2 teaspoon honey
1/4 teaspoon sea salt
1/4 teaspoon black pepper

4 cups loosely packed mixed leafy baby greens
  such as arugula or baby spinach
olive oil spray
1 tablespoon sesame seeds
1/4 teaspoon crushed red pepper
1 tablespoon finely chopped fresh sage (optional)

Simply spray the lettuce leaves with olive oil and gently toss the remaining ingredients. Can be served hot or cold. Make it a meal by adding shrimp, white fish, salmon, or chicken breast.

Slimming Sauces and Thermogenic Dressings

Anyone can cook using butter and fats, but it's an art to cook lean and clean. All it takes is a little creativity and a few old Italian tricks. Your taste buds will adapt to not using butter and using less oil after a while. And you won't even notice that these delicious sauces are low- or no-fat. Most of the time, it's the sauce you crave, not what's underneath it. You'll be surprised how much your whole family will love these finger-licking good sauces.

These dressings are just as delicious and great for making any kind of salad. Think out of the box when it comes to mixing tuna or salmon, shrimp, seafood, crab, chicken, or all vegetables salads if you're in a pinch. Don't underestimate those bagged lettuces when you're tight on time and your store's salad bar offers pick-up ready veggies for you to dunk. How easy is that for a weekday snack that boosts you metabolism and causes weight loss?

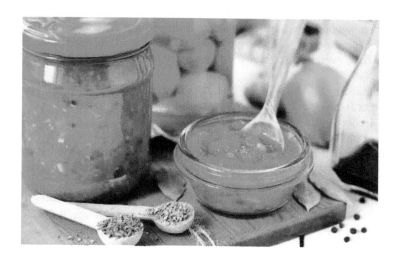

Melt-Fat Marinara

Minutes to Prepare: 5 ◆ Minutes to Cook: 10 ◆ Number of Servings: 4, if you're lucky

This is a must-have for all refrigerators, so plan on cooking this every Sunday night to use all week on top of your lean proteins and vegetables. My favorite thing is when my kids walk into the house and say "Wow! What's for dinner?" when they smell it cooking. We can practically drink this sauce, and kids love to dunk their food into it—makes healthy food fun. Melt-Fat Marinara is an awesome topping for any and all foods—even as a salad dressing. It's is a great source of lycopene that's good for health because it doesn't contain the salt and sugar ketchup does. Retrain your whole house to use this instead; it's fresher and has a more gourmet feel, even when served at picnics and barbeques. Play with it by adding your own fresh herbs and buying different typed of tomato sizes and brands and you'll have your one signature must-have sauce—or gravy as we Italians call it.

16 oz. can of crushed tomatoes with basil, oregano,
    garlic, and onions already mixed in for convenience
2 tablespoon fat free chicken broth, IF needed for
    a thinner sauce-less for thicker

1 teaspoon olive oil
1 tablespoon minced garlic or 1 garlic clove minced
olive oil spray if needed.

Lightly sauté garlic in olive oil. Remove pan from heat. Add crushed tomatoes and return to medium heat, then simmer.

When cooking with less oil, watch food carefully as it may burn quickly. You can always add water or fat-free chicken broth to rehydrate if needed. There's no need to add more oil.

No-Cook Fast and Easy Tomato Sauce

Minutes to Prepare: 2 ◆ Number of Servings: 2 to 3

Want faster sauce? Try my no-cook tomato sauce. This sauce is awesome especially when you have fresh tomatoes from the garden or you need a quick, delicious sauce to top off your clean foods. Get creative and try using all different kinds of tomatoes or whatever you have on hand. Add chopped onion or a dash of wine vinegar for a pop. Enjoy it hot or cold, even as a soup. Just add water or fat-free chicken broth.

1 pint cherry or grape tomatoes
garlic as desired (minced or fresh-your call)
fresh basil or dried basil (if desired)

spray olive oil
salt and pepper to taste

Roughly chop the tomatoes and place in bowl. Stir in basil, spray with olive oil, salt, and pepper. Allow to marinate 10 minutes if you can stand to wait to dig in. Otherwise, you're ready to go.

No time to make either sauce? Use your favorite salsa on top of your lean protein or over vegetables for a fast delicious alternative. Still, nothing beats God's fresh ingredients and you'll be a superstar at home with these.

Top Secret Tuna Sauce
(The Vegetarian Meat Sauce)

Minutes to Prepare: 5 ◆ Minutes to Cook: 15 to 20 ◆ Number of Servings: 2

I know, I know… Tuna in a sauce? Trust me on this one, you are going to want to try this secret slimming sauce because it is delicious. This was my Aunt Rosemary's mom's recipe and I couldn't believe it was tuna when I tried it for the first time. Adding tuna to your sauce not only makes it tastier, but it also makes it healthier. Tuna doesn't only thicken, it is one of the world's healthiest foods as it contains a rare form of selenium which plays a role as an important antioxidant binding together with mercury compounds and thus lowering the risk of mercury problems. The fact that Tuna contains all of the essential amino acids as well as Omega-3's gives you a good reason to eat it, not to mention that eating seafood helps you lose weight faster. And guess what the #1 fish most people will eat? Tuna. It's lower in fat than chicken and turkey, and contains 34 micrograms of iodine per 6-ounce can. Iodine, by the way, has been known to play a key role in boosting your metabolism. Finally, don't let all the mercury stories scare you. If you're eating a balanced diet, consuming 1 to 2 cans per week is fine. Did you know that most mercury poisoning comes from buying cheap Omega-3 supplements? Psst. Don't tell your non-fish eating kids and be sure to hide the cans of tuna; they will never know and love this sauce.

1 (6 1/2) oz. can tuna	1/2 medium onion, chopped
1 small can of plum tomatoes	1 tablespoon olive oil
1 tablespoon fat-free chicken broth	1 garlic clove crushed or 1 tablespoon minced garlic
Pepper	3 anchovy fillets (optional)

Heat oil in frying pan, add onions and sauté 5 minutes (add some broth if needed). Add garlic and cook until onions start to brown. Add anchovies if desired (crush them with spoon).

Add tomatoes, simmer covered to form a sauce about 15 minutes.

Drain the tuna and break into large flakes. Add tuna to sauce with a little pepper (anchovies and tuna are already salty). Simmer, uncovered, for 5 minutes. Juices will evaporate and sauce will thicken.

This recipe can be made with boiled shrimp or clams so get creative and leave the fattening meats out of it.

HERB SAUCE

Minutes to Prepare: 5 to 10 ◆ Minutes to Cook: 5 ◆ Number of Servings: 2 to 4

I come from an Italian family that can cook, but they never learned how to cook lean. I adore food—especially Italian food—so I took the time to travel in the Mediterranean to learn their way of cooking, which is the healthiest way to live lean for life. It was during my travels to Sicily that I learned how to make this herb sauce. It's more delicious than it sounds and goes great on top of fish and chicken or as a dipping sauce for vegetables. Try it and I'm sure you'll love it, too. What makes this recipe unique is that it uses minimal oil, no butter, and is meat-, gluten-, and soy-free. It's free of just about everything except good taste.

2 oz. anchovies mashed	1 tablespoon capers
1/2 to 1 cup of chopped mushrooms	2 tablespoon parsley, chopped
2 garlic cloves, chopped	4 to 5 large basil leaves (chopped)
1/2 tsp hot pepper flakes	1/3 cup of fat-free chicken broth
olive oil spray	

Mix all ingredients together, cook over low heat to warm up slowly. Stir and keep hot. Pour over fish, chicken, or your favorite vegetables.

This recipes is originally prepared with 1/4 cup of black olives, 1/4 cup of green olives, and 1/3 cup of olive oil. My family doesn't like olives and I don't need the excess fat. Feel free to prepare it the way your family likes it best, and be prepared for a wild ride of flavor as this recipe will dazzle your taste buds.

PESTO
(PREPARE-TO-BOOST-YOUR-METABOLISM PESTO)

Minutes to Prepare: 5 ◆ Number of Servings: 2 to 4

Everyone loves a good pesto sauce, but it's more fattening than a cheeseburger and French fries. There are many different ways to make it, but only this recipe is clean enough to help you get lean. Take the time to play with this recipe and make it yours—that's the secret to living lean. This sauce can be stored in a jar in a refrigerator for several weeks by adding more broth or a little olive oil to coat the top of the pesto. It's perfect for when you need a change from red sauce and it doesn't have to be cooked if you're in a rush.

1 cup fresh basil leaves, packed
1/4 cup of grated Italian cheese (look for low-fat)
1 cut fat-free chicken broth

4 garlic cloves
1 cup of parsley, packed
1/8 cup pignoli nuts (optional; omit if trying to lose weight)

Place all ingredients in a blender and blend together using low speed with 1/2 cup of fat free broth. Stop every few seconds to scrape the sides of the blender down until everything is evenly mixed.
   Blend remaining 1/2 cup fat free broth in a steady stream. Continue blending until smooth in consistency.
   Pour over fish or chicken or use a vegetable dip.

BELL PEPPER COULIS SAUCE

Minutes to Prepare: 10 ◆ Minutes to Cook: 20 ◆ Makes 1 Pint

What's Coulis? Pronounced "koo-lee," it is a simple sauce made of pureed vegetables which can be served hot or cold. This recipe for bell pepper coulis is great for company or on a hot night. Coulis makes a great veggie dip that's almost calorie- free so you can dip shrimp and vegetables all night. It can be made with red, yellow, or even orange peppers (not green) and makes a great soup hot or cold. This simple slimming sauce is one of my family's favorites and is very versatile—perfect poured over roasted vegetables, shrimp, any white fish, and, of course, chicken. This metabolic-boosting coulis is fast and easy to make and superhealthy, loaded with vitamins A and C.

2 to 3 large red, yellow, or orange bell peppers
1/4 cup vegetable stock or vegetable bouillon
sea salt & pepper to taste
   (white pepper is awesome in this recipe)

2 OZ fat-free chicken broth or extra-virgin olive oil
Tablespoon Balsamic Vinegar
2 tablespoons chopped shallots (optional)

Remove core, seeds, and membranes from the peppers and roughly chop them.
   Add broth and heat in a sauté pan over medium heat for 1 to 2 minutes. Add shallots if using and sauté until they are slightly translucent.
   Reduce heat to low, add the chopped pepper. Cover and sweat for about 15 minutes or until tender.
   Add a couple of tablespoons of stock and cook for another 1 to 2 minutes. Remove from heat and puree in blender. Caution: Be careful when blending hot liquids in blender as steam may pop lid off blender. Start on slow

speed with lid ajar slowly increasing blender speed.

Add vinegar. Adjust consistency with remaining stock and season to taste with salt and pepper.

Mustard sauce and dressing
(AKA Metabolic boosting Mustard sauce)

Minutes to Prepare: 5♦ Minutes to Cook: 5 ♦ Serves: 4 to 6

While mustard sauce is usually a cream sauce, this one is lean, clean, and oh-so-delicious. It's awesome with eggs or over vegetables, fish, or chicken, and makes an awesome salad dressing. I learned about this sauce/dressing from my bodybuilder friends who live to be lean and will not eat fatty foods (that's why they are so lean). Tangy mustard sauce has practically no fat or carbs and is low-sodium to boot. Bodybuilders are very creative when it comes to food because their meals are so precious so they make sure they enjoy what they are eating.

olive oil spray
2 minced garlic cloves or store bought
1/4 cup balsamic or red wine vinegar
1/4 cup fat-free, low-sodium chicken broth
salt and pepper to taste

2 tablespoon prepared mustard-of choice (Dijon is best)
3/4 teaspoon chopped rosemary (optional)

Spray pan with olive oil over medium heat. Add minced garlic and sauté 30 seconds, stirring constantly.

Stir in vinegar, broth, and Dijon mustard. Bring to boil. Cook until reduced to 1/4 cup (about 5 minutes), stirring occasionally. Stir in rosemary and black pepper.

For a really special day add 2 tablespoons maple syrup for extra yumminess.

Tangy Mustard Dressing

Need a delicious salad dressing when you're out with friends? This salad dressing is the easiest and most delicious. Best of all, it can be made anywhere, anytime—even at a diner. Simply mix together mustard and vinegar (anything you can get your hands on) and add 1 packet of Equal, if needed. Salt and pepper to taste. Voila! You have a delicious fat-free dressing. No more excuses.

TOP FIVE Ways to Eat Your Veggies
1) Chopped salads or veggies already cut up, prewashed salad, or slaw style.
2) Dunked raw.
3) Cut head of lettuce in 1/2 and grill it and top with dressing
4) As soup. Just add water and your favorite seasoning
5) Pureed and added to your favorite sauce or dressing to thicken it—not your waist.

Sexy Salsa Dressing

Minutes to Prepare: 15 ♦ Minutes to Cook: 20 ♦ Serves: 6

This simple dressing is not simple when it comes to taste and the big bang it packs in flavor. Use it on salads, over fish, or as a stir-fry mix in. Always remember you can dip boring veggies or dull, dry lean protein in these dressings making the more appealing. Everyone loves fondue style. Sexy salsa is great as a salad dressing-makes a great sauce for shrimp salad and or dip. I think every refrigerator should have a stash of this----it's delicious and kids love to help make it too.

4 large ripe tomatoes, cut into bite sized pieces
1 large green bell pepper, cut into bite-sized pieces
1 large red bell pepper, cut into bite sized pieces
1/2 sweet red onions chopped
1/2 tsp NoSalt to taste

1 bunch cilantro, stems cut off and leaves coarsely chopped
3 green onions, chopped
1 lime juiced

In a large salad bowl, lightly mix the tomatoes, cilantro, green and red bell peppers, green onions, and sweet red onion until thoroughly combined. Squeeze lime juice over salad. Sprinkle with salt to serve.

Can't make it fast enough? Use canned chopped tomatoes. And if you like it hotter, add finely chopped jalapenos.

Thai Dipping sauce or Salad Dressing

Minutes to Prepare: 5 ♦ Minutes to Cook: 5 ♦ Serves: 2

This sauce will get your kids and whole family to devour whatever healthy food you're trying to disguise. I'll let you in on a little secret: I hated vegetables until I realized that eating them helped me lose weight and I hated the fact that my plate was bare unless I filled it with veggies. The secret to my vegetable eating success is finding delicious, creative ways to enjoy them. This is one of my favorites and it goes great on chicken or as a salad dressing—it's especially good for dipping. My kids love dunking snap peas in it. Make extra as you won't be able to keep it in the house very long. Even veggies sent to school in a lunch box will get eaten. I always take this dipping sauce and vegetables to picnics or any outing that may not be particularly healthy so I have something delicious to eat. Guess what? Everyone wants my food. Serve this one hot or cold (It does contain a little bit of soy sauce but not enough to wreck your diet and you're eating cleaner so you have budget for it)

2 tablespoons PB2 peanut butter powder*
1 tablespoon water
1/4 teaspoon pepper (ground is best)
1/8 teaspoon sesame oil

1 tablespoon low-sodium soy sauce
1/8 teaspoon garlic powder
1 teaspoon Splenda brown sugar
1/8 teaspoon Szechwan chili sauce (optional)

Blend all ingredients well and serve. Refrigerate any remaining sauce. How easy is that?

*PB2 by Bell Plantation (bellplantation.com) is a peanut butter powder available in many stores and online.

Be LEAN Blue Cheese

Minutes to Prepare: 5 ◆ Serves: 4 to 6 salads

We all need help when it comes to enjoying clean food, and blue cheese is a helper that just about everyone loves, especially for veggie dipping, on top of dry turkey burgers, or simply drizzled on grilled romaine lettuce (my favorite) for a fast, easy, weight-loss friendly, and scrumptious salad. However, blue cheese also dumps about 30 grams of fat on your salad (because it contains oil, mayonnaise, cheese, and buttermilk), which puts you well over the 15 to 20 grams of fat you need to stay under when trying to lose weight. Here is an easy version anyone can make, and while it's not the leanest and cleanest (it does contain some dairy), it will still keep you out of the real stuff, saving you lots of fat and calories. When you crave certain foods but want to behave, remember, it's all about replacing the food with healthier version so you can live life lean even as your metabolism slows down. You won't even know it's healthy. My family hasn't figured it out yet. This dressing is also great on top of Turkey burgers, Portobello mushroom burgers or dip chicken on a skewer instead of fattening wings. Grab your celery and get ready to dunk. WARNING: Buy extra vegetables to dip; they will disappear faster than ever.

1/4 cup blue cheese finely chopped
juice of 1/2 lemon (try it with a Meyer lemon)
1 tablespoon white vinegar
1/4 teaspoon salt
black pepper to taste
sprinkle of onion powder

1/2 cup Greek yogurt (look for the lowest calorie and zero fat one you can find at your local store) for a thicker dressing or you can use buttermilk for lighter version that's thinner
sprinkle of garlic powder
dash of Equal or Splenda.

Finely chop and break apart blue cheese into tiny crumbles. Combine blue cheese, Greek yogurt, lemon juice, and vinegar in a bowl (better yet make it in a jar so you can save the remaining dressing for later) and mix well.

Add all of the other seasonings and stir well with fork until cheese is no longer clumping up. The secret to disguising this health version is to make sure its mixed well.

You can adjust to desired thickness by using thicker yogurts, or if you prefer it thinner add water (1 tablespoon at a time) until you reach the desired thickness you prefer. On special occasions, try a drizzle of honey in it. Want more pizzazz? Add a dash of hot sauce; it's practically calorie-free.

Fat-Blasting Cesar Dressing

Minutes to Prepare: 5 ◆ Serves: 4 to 6 salads

Who doesn't adore Caesar dressing? I could live on Caesar salads every day, and I did at first. This was one of my big mistakes when I started eating healthy and found I still wasn't losing weight. You know why? Depending on what you put in your salad, it can have more calories than a cheeseburger and fries combined. I spent my life researching ways to make recipes leaner, but leaner without tasting yummy wasn't good enough. I picked the brains of the chefs at Martha Stewart's and asked all of my chef friends (while waiting on TV sets I am in the back room picking brains of awesome people like Chef Big Daddy Aaron McCargo, Jr.) to find out their secrets and came up with this fast and easy lean Caesar dressing. If you're pressed for time, you could use the lowest-calorie bottled Caesar dressing you can find in your store, but there is nothing like making this from scratch. This recipe is egg-less and can be drizzled on top of your fish or shrimp, or used as a dipping sauce. In my house it's all about the dunk. You can eat it every day if it helps you reach your veggie quota. Don't tell anyone, but I bring my own stash when I'm eating out and want to enjoy my meal without breaking my plan. Just be prepared to share—everyone always uses mine up.

1/3 cup grated Parmesan cheese
(I prefer Parmigiano Reggiano)
1/2 teaspoon Dijon mustard
1 tablespoon fat-free chicken broth or if you can
    afford the calories, 1 tablespoon extra-virgin
    olive oil

1/4 fresh lemon juice (Meyer lemons make it better)
1 small garlic clove
2 anchovy fillets*
5 tablespoons fat-free plain Greek yogurt
(lowest calorie you can find)

In a food processor add the cheese, lemon juice, garlic clove, Dijon mustard, and the anchovies.

Blend in food processor for 15 to 20 seconds. Add the oil and yogurt and blend for additional 15 seconds and there you have it. Hold the croutons.

*Not an anchovy fan? Leave them out, but they are what make this dressing so awesome.

GREEN AND LEAN CUCUMBER RANCH DRESSING

Minutes to Prepare: 10 ◆ Serves: 6 salads

Ranch is one of the most popular dressings in the United States, a staple at every salad bar. But it is horrible for you, unless you eat this green and lean version. Kids love it and moms approve—and so will your skinny jeans. Unlike other ranch dressings that contain everything that's bad for you, This version is light and very refreshing thanks to the thermogenic cucumbers that help blast the metabolism and keep calories low. It will lure you into eating more salads and veggies. Even fussy eaters crave this one.

1/2 cup low-fat buttermilk
1 small cucumber, peeled and seeds removed
    (you can leave seeds in for texture-I do)
3 tablespoons fresh or dried parsley
juice of 1/2 a lemon
Salt and pepper to taste

1/4 cup fat free plain Greek yogurt (look for the lowest
    calorie and fat at your supermarket)
1 clove of garlic
1/4 scallions (optional)
1/8 teaspoon garlic powder

Combine all ingredients in a blender or food processor and blend for 15 to 30 seconds until desired consistency is reached.

For extra oomph, add a dash of horseradish.

HALLELUJAH HONEY MUSTARD, THE SIMPLEST SKINNY DRESSING EVER

Minutes to Prepare: 10 ◆ Serves: 1 to 2 salads

Honey mustard has always been one of my favorites, naturally because it's sweet. This dressing is delicious and good for you—not to mention it's fast and easy and kills the bottled stuff you can buy. Kids love it and will eat their veggies and chicken if you make this dunk sauce. I love it after a day in the country with the kids when we pick up a local bottle of honey and fresh vegetables at a farm stand. It's amazing how the small things like this can motivate kids to eat healthfully. Get them involved and make a day of learning about honey and what makes it different when it's from your local area. They will be fascinated and want to eat it. Did you know pure honey is antibacterial and antifungal; helps reduce coughs and throat irritations, and may ease gastric intestinal disorders? Don't forget though that honey is a sugar, and all sugar can elevate blood sugar levels no matter how healthy it is.

It is a good idea to include honey with a protein to help blunt blood sugar levels form rising or you can always take a Carb Edge to keep sugar levels in line. Try to eat this on the weekends to keep things balanced.

1 tablespoon Dijon mustard
1 teaspoon honey

Mix together and eat.

Want it sugar free? Add a dash of water to thin out and add 1 packet of Splenda for a sugar free version.

If you need a bigger batch for company, add buttermilk (skim milk works, too). Adjust the mustard to honey to taste as desired. If you want a thicker version, process some radishes in a food processor and they will thicken it right up without anyone even knowing you added them. Radishes, by the way, are virtually calorie-free.

MOJITO LIME DRESSING

Minutes to Prepare: 5 ◆ Serves: 4

This is delicious on a hot summer night on just about anything from salads to a dip for veggies to topping for your Lean Tuna Burgers. It has a little nonfat mayo in it, and when I make it I use it sparingly if at all, saving the full mayonnaise amount for special occasions. Try this when you need a change over your salad or mix cabbage or broccoli (try pre-shredded store-bought bags when you're in a hurry) with it for a delicious lime slaw.

1/2 cup fat-free mayonnaise   2 tablespoons chopped mint
1 tablespoon fresh lime juice (bottled is OK, too)

Combine ingredients and stir until blended.

MELT-FAT MEDITERRANEAN

Minutes to Prepare: 5 ◆ Serves: 1

This dressing is a classic all across the Mediterranean, but it only becomes lean when you reduce olive oil amounts or better yet use spray olive oil instead so you can portion control. Melt-Fat Mediterranean dressing is simply delicious and a great way to show off the taste of fresh vegetables and seafood—the cleaner the food the better. It goes with everything. Just be careful with the olive oil and you'll be fine.

1 teaspoon high-quality extra-virgin olive oil (look for cold-pressed) or olive oil spray for better portion control

dash sea salt and pepper

juice from one lemon (Meyer lemons make it extra special)

sprinkle of lemon zest

Simply mix everything together and use this to dress your salads and other cooking needs. It is the simplest dressing ever and the best tasting.

> **When all else fails, go for your favorite bottled dressing from your local supermarket. Mine is Paul Newman's. To make it leaner, I dilute it with vinegar to reduce the fat and salt. Always look for a bottle with the lowest calories, carbohydrates, and salt you can find. And don't ever forget to be on the lookout for sugar. Yes, dressings can be full of it.**

THE BEST TO-GO ON-THE-GO MEALS

Whether you're an office worker, student, or a harried mom running around to doctor's appointments and school meetings, most lunchtimes (or meals on the go) consist of being held hostage to a handful of fast-food and sit-down chains. This is exactly why the Complete Protein Shake makes losing weight so easy. All you have to do is drink your nutrition and go on with your day. But brown-bagging it is inevitable at times whether you're with family at the beach, in your backyard by the pool, or at ball game: You need to be ready with the right foods. Lunch or any meal on the go still needs to consist of a small serving of lean protein and vegetables if you're serious about boosting your metabolism. Try these fast easy, grab-and-go lunches (when you can't drink a shake or eat a Lean Bar), and you'll never be caught downing a drive-thru milkshake for lunch again.

1) Make lettuce wraps instead of using bread. Simply wrap your favorite protein in a lettuce leaf. It's what celebs do.
2) Make it a salad (vegetable salads too) of course without all the croutons, cheese, bacon, yolks, beans, or full-fat dressings.
3) Slim down and fill up with soup. Soup can be enjoyed hot or cold depending on the season.

It's easy to make Lean Light salads. Simply combine tuna, egg whites, chicken, salmon or sliced turkey from the deli—works in a pinch. All of these ingredients can be mixed with the dressings in this book.

If you're really in a rush, try these simpler varieties:

1) Start with a lettuce wrap, a base of lettuces leaves chopped up, or you can use your favorite vegetables if you prefer—as long as you don't use bread. Simply mix the items below with one of the thermogenic dressings on page 243 or use a simple store-bought fat-free mustard, salsa, or the cleanest bottled dressing you can find. Remember to look for fat-free or the lowest fat available, low or no carbs, little or no sugar (yes dressings have sugar in them), and of course low sodium.
2) Lean Protein: Tuna, salmon, chicken breast, crab meat, egg whites, or 2 to 3 slices of low-sodium deli turkey.
3) Mix-ins: Add your favorite fat-free salsa, Dijon mustard, or any fat-free mustard
   - Add 1/2 to 1 cup of your favorite frozen mixed veggies and season with Mrs. Dash, McCargo's Signature Blend, or your favorite seasoning.
   - Add fresh lemon juice, Dijon mustard, and garlic paste (made by finely chopping a fresh clove and smashing it into a paste), and season with fresh pepper. Mix veggie/tuna mixture together until well incorporated. Taste. Add salt if necessary.
   - Add crunchy veggies like carrots, celery, onion, or think out of the box and add pineapple chunks or apple chunks to your chicken salads.

MORE SLIMMING SALADS

BLUE CHEESE BLUES: Slice a head of iceberg lettuce in half and drizzle with BE Lean Blue cheese over the big chunk. ◆ THAI: Buy a container of your favorite greens and 3 ounces of chicken breast (canned is fine) drizzle with Thai salad dressing and top with a few slivered almonds. Great with chopped scallions. ◆ CAESAR: Toss 3 cups of romaine with shrimp or salmon or chicken breast. ◆ SEXY SALSA SALAD: This is a great chopped salad. Chop 3 cups of your favorite lettuce and 3 ounces of shrimp or chicken chunks and toss with Sexy Salsa dressing. ◆ FAJITA SALAD: Make lean fajitas (sauté 3 oz. cooked chicken breast with assorted peppers, salt, pepper, and olive oil spray) and top your salad. No dressing needed. Let the juices drip onto the salad.

SNEAK IN A LITTLE COMPLETE PROTEIN POWDER TO BOOST YOUR METABOLISM

POWER YOUR METABOLISM WITH PROTEIN PANCAKES

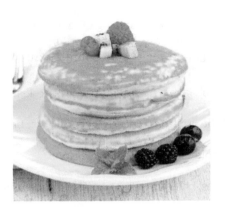

2 scoops of your favorite flavor of Complete Protein powder
1/8 cup of water

Place Complete Protein powder in a bowl and add just enough water that the mixture has a consistency similar to pancake batter (it should be slightly lumpy). Pour the mixture into a nonstick skillet sprayed with nonstick cooking spray, and cook on medium heat, 1 to 2 minutes each side. Top with cinnamon or 0-calorie syrup of your choice. (I like Walden's.) Try experimenting with vanilla, almond, or coconut extracts to get lots of flavor without the calories.

WARM METABOLIC DRINKS

You can mix these in a blender or use a frother for a real treat.
SKINNY HOT CHOCOLATE: Add 1 to 2 scoops of chocolate Complete Protein powder to warm (not hot water, it will cause shake to curdle) water.
LEAN LATTE: Add 1 to 2 Scoops of vanilla Complete Protein powder to 6 oz. warm coffee and sprinkle with cinnamon.
METABOLIC MOCCAHCCINO: Add 1 to 2 scoops of your favorite Complete Protein powder to 6 oz. of warm coffee.
HOT PEPPERMINT MOCHA: Add 1 to 2 scoops of chocolate Complete Protein powder and 3 drops of mint extract to 6 oz. of warm coffee.
WARM ALMOND AB BLAST: Add 1 to 2 scoops of vanilla or chocolate Complete Protein powder and 3 drops of almond extract to 6 oz. of warm coffee.

TURBO-CHARGING PROTEIN-PACKED JELL-O

2 scoops of your favorite Complete Protein powder
1 package sugar free Jell-O (any flavor)

Make Jell-O according to directions. Before setting to gel, add protein powder. Let stand to set. I always have this on hand so I can CHOW whenever you need to.

TRY THESE FLAVOR BOOSTERS

Adding flavor doesn't mean you need to add calories. Try experimenting with the following flavor boosters for a calorie-free flavor punch.

EXTRACTS: Vanilla, Almond, Coconut, Banana, Mint.

PEANUT BUTTER: Add a teaspoon to satisfy your craving.

SUGAR-FREE FAT-FREE JELL-O: Try every flavor under the sun until you fall in love with one. My favorite flavor is lemon.

COOKIES FOR WEIGHT LOSS

2 scoops of your favorite Complete Protein Powder
1 egg white

Mix egg white and protein powder in bowl. Add water to the mixture until it forms a doughy substance. Spray a bowl with nonstick cooking spray and add batter. Place in a microwave and heat 15 to 45 seconds, depending on the power of your microwave.

QUICK AND EASY SLIMMING COOKIES: Don't feel like messing up you kitchen? Cut up pieces of a Lean Bar and place on dish sprayed with nonstick cooking spray. Microwave for 2 to 40 seconds, depending on the power of your microwave. Cool slightly. Sprinkle with cinnamon and enjoy.

I WANNA BE LEAN ICE CREAM

There are thousands of options to choose from when it comes to making lean ice cream. Choose the flavor you're craving and enjoy. (P.S. They make great shakes, too)

PEANUT BUTTER AND CHOCOLATE DREAM

1 to 2 scoops of chocolate Complete Protein powder
1 teaspoon peanut butter
1/2 cup water
4 ice cubes.
Fill food processor with water and ice cubes and blend until the ice is crushed into a fine snow. Scrape down sides of processor. Add Complete Protein and peanut butter. Mix for 2 to 3 minutes. Then serve and enjoy.

STRAWBERRY TRUFFLE ICE CREAM

2 scoops strawberry Complete Protein powder
3 teaspoons sugar-free white chocolate pudding mix
1/2 cup water
4 ice cubes
Fill food processor with water and ice cubes and blend until the ice is crushed into a fine snow. Scrape down sides of processor. Add Complete Protein and white chocolate pudding mix. Process for 2 to 3 minutes. Then serve and enjoy.

VERY VANILLA ICE CREAM

2 scoops vanilla Complete Protein powder
1 1/2 envelopes of unflavored gelatin
1/4 cup cold water
1teaspoon vanilla extract
3/4 boiling water
Sprinkle gelatin over cold water to soften. Add vanilla and boiling water. Stir to dissolve gelatin. Refrigerate until mixture starts to set. Mix at high speed until mixture becomes frothy. Add Complete Protein and beat at high speed for 10 minutes. Pour into 2 one-pint plastic containers and freeze.

DECADENT DESSERTS

Are you like me, do you live for dessert? I am more than willing to give up the carbs; I think they are sadly overrated. But I cannot imagine living without dessert. The good news: You don't have to. *The Metabolism Solution* is specifically designed to boost your metabolism so you burn more calories even at rest which leaves some room in your caloric budget for Real Life Indulgences—for those moments when you just have to have something delicious. Dessert is why we drink the shake in the morning—it allows us a little room for real life.

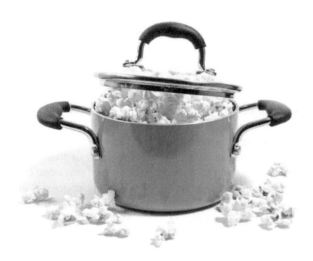

KETTLE CORN

Minutes to Prepare: 5 ◆ Minutes to Cook: 5 ◆ Number of Servings: 2 ◆ Serving Size: 3 Cups

I live for sweets. I don't mind eating really lean all day if I know I can have this as a snack later on. I know we shouldn't eat at night, but the truth is I do. I find it easiest to resist temptation all day and then allow myself what I crave at night. Popcorn is a whole grain and full of fiber. Add some Complete Protein powder to it and you have a terrific metabolic-boosting, faster-fat-burning snack. Its sweet and salty flavors work for just about everyone. If you don't have the time to make your own kettle corn, look for the cleanest one (lowest fat and sugars possible) you can find at your local grocery store. If you are one of the lucky ones lacking a sweet tooth, try one of the other varieties below.

6 cups air-popped popcorn or whatever popped corn you have

1/8 tsp. NoSalt or salt substitute (Can't find one? Use salt.)

2 packets of Stevia, Splenda, or your
    personal favorite sweetener

butter-flavored cooking spray

Combine ingredients in a bowl. With back of a teaspoon, crush mixture until it is like powder. Doing this makes it easier to sprinkle and the salt isn't as concentrated. Try whirring the seasonings in a food processor to crush into smaller particles and then store them in a shaker for faster, easier use.

When your corn is finished popping, give it a spray with butter-flavored cooking spray and quickly sprinkle your homemade kettle corn seasoning. Toss the corn until seasoning is evenly distributed.

MORE FLAVORS
CINNAMON SUGAR: Add 1/4 teaspoon cinnamon
CHOCOLATE POPCORN: Add 1 teaspoon to 1 tablespoon chocolate Complete Protein powder
PIZZA POPCORN: Add desired amount of grated parmesan cheese, 1 teaspoon dried oregano, 1 tablespoon finely chopped sun-dried tomatoes, 1/4 teaspoon red pepper flakes, 1/4 garlic powder

PROTEIN PEANUT BUTTER BLISS BALLS

Minutes to Prepare: 5 ◆ Minutes to Cook: 10 ◆ Serving Size: 1 ball

This has got to be one of the best weekend cheat foods on the planet. Thank God I don't have time to make this often, but when I do, I am sure to make extra and freeze them for those need-one-now moments. (Don't we all have them?) They are easy to prepare and healthy enough to eat when you need a fix. This should make enough servings to last a couple of weeks. Store the remainder in a Tupperware container in the fridge. Remember, this is a weekend cheat food, unless you can only eat one. These peanut butter balls are rich in calories, but the whey gives you high-quality protein, the oats give you fiber and low-glycemic carbs, the honey boosts your immune system, and the peanut butter provides healthy unsaturated fats and antioxidants. Want to go really clean? Skip the oats.

2 scoops LynFit chocolate or vanilla
    Complete Protein powder
1 cup natural peanut butter

1/4 cup honey
3/4 cup raw oats

Mix all the ingredients in a large bowl. Powder your hands with some flour (to prevent stickiness) and form into 1-inch balls and place on a baking sheet. Bake at 374 degrees for 5 to 10 minutes.

For a special occasion treat: Dip them in melted dark chocolate and roll them in shredded coconut, sprinkles, or nuts. They make great gifts.

RICH COCOA SORBETO

Minutes to Prepare: 10 ◆ Minutes to Freeze: 20 ◆ Serving: 4

One thing we all crave at one time or another is ice cream. Why? It's mood food. Ice cream is one of the biggest diet destroyers. To help you get your fix without sabotaging all the work you do on The Metabolism Solution *plan, I created this sorbeto that, unlike ice cream, isn't loaded with fat or sugar so it's low in calories and carbs. My sorbeto has 1 gram of fat and 25 carbs. You can keep losing weight even if you eat it—dare I say it—every day? You can thank researchers in part for removing some of the guilt from this guilty pleasure. Studies have shown that chocolate, particularly dark chocolate with at least 70 percent cocoa, can help protect you from heart disease and some cancers while boosting your immune system thanks to plant chemicals called flavonoids. Ounce for ounce, cocoa powder has the highest concentration of age-fighting antioxidants than other foods. Most chocolate desserts are loaded with sugar, heavy cream, butter, and other heavy ingredients that neutralize cocoa's healthy effects. Not this one.*

1 cup natural cocoa powder
3/4 honey (substitute with 3/4 cup Splenda
    or Stevia for even cleaner version)
1 1/2 teaspoon vanilla extract

1 3/4 cups of water
1/2 teaspoon salt

Place cocoa into small sauce pan. Slowly whisk in 3/4 cup water until cocoa is dissolved and there are no lumps.

Whisk in honey or sweetener used, salt, and remaining 1 cup water. Stir over medium heat until mixture begins to boil. Remove from heat. Stir in vanilla.

When cool, pour mixture into the canister of ice cream maker, freeze according to manufacturer's instructions or you can freeze mixture in a bowl, then process in a food processor, and re-freeze until sorbet is set.

My trick? Add 1 cup of chocolate Complete Protein powder in place of the cocoa to help keep your metabolism revved—it makes it even yummier.

Not a chocolate fan? Try these recipes instead.

STRAWBERRIES AND CREAM: Replace the cocoa with 1/2 cup of strawberry Complete Protein power and 1/2 cup vanilla Complete Protein.
VERY VANILLA SORBETO: Use 1 cup of vanilla Complete Protein powder instead of cocoa.

Any of the Shake recipes (p. 47) that you love can also be made into sorbet. Simply freeze them. Allow them to thaw just enough so you can easily eat them with a spoon. Customer favorites? Cookies and Cream, Creamsicle, and Banana Cream. Create some tartness with lemon juice or use Jell-O powder or extracts for flavor. You can experiment using anything that doesn't add calories to the recipe so you don't have to limit this to the weekends.

ROCKY ROAD HIGH PROTEIN FUDGE BARS

Minutes to Prepare: 10 ◆ Minutes to Freeze: 20 ◆ Serving: TK

Your new favorite, healthy "cheat day" dessert. This "fudge" is full of lean protein, fiber, and calcium; honey is great for B vitamins and boosting your immunity. You'll never eat regular fudge again. Make extra for when your sweet tooth calls.

1 cup chocolate Complete Protein powder
1/4 to 1/2 cup marshmallows
1/4 cup rolled oats

1/2 cup Nutella Spread
1/4 cup honey (Substitute 1/4 cup
   Stevia or Splenda if desired)

Equipment Needed:
10 pieces aluminum foil sized 1/2 roll x 6 inches
Blender
Heavy spatula

Freezer or ice pack
Bowl

In a large mixing bowl, blend rolled oats (uncooked), 1 cup chocolate LynFit Complete Protein powder until blended.

Add Nutella and honey and mix until thoroughly blended and it holds its shape. Add marshmallows until desired look and taste is met.

Form a patty one-inch thick or make a candy-bar shape using the spatula and place on aluminum foil. Put in freezer and chill until frozen.

When nicely frozen, remove and cut into smaller bars of desired size. Keep chilled until just before eating if possible so the cold bars and patties keep their shape (and it keeps them from going bad).

Variations:
- Add one banana to the mixture to make the texture chewier
- Add dry spices such as cinnamon and nutmeg
- Add walnuts or almonds
- Add a shot of coconut or vanilla flavoring (add extra oats to compensate for added liquid)

APPLE WHEY GOOD CRISPILICIOUS

Minutes to Prepare: 10 ◆ Minutes to Cook: 20 to 30 ◆ Servings: 4

Great to have on hand when company is coming. The vanilla Complete Protein powder adds a metabolic-boosting protein punch. This dessert has fiber to help keep things regular and apples have been known to "suppress" appetite. Keep plenty of apples on hand so you are never without. Use this recipe when your cravings are pushing you to go off, but you're still inside the guard rail. It won't stop the fat-loss process. An apple a day keeps the pounds away.

BASE
3 apples, cored and sliced
1 1/2 teaspoon lemon juice
1 scoop vanilla Complete Protein powder
1/2 teaspoon cinnamon

1/2 cup applesauce, unsweetened
1 teaspoon Splenda
1 teaspoon Splenda brown sugar

TOPPING
1 cup oatmeal
1 scoop vanilla Complete Protein powder

2 tablespoons Splenda brown sugar
2 tablespoons Smart Balance (optional; you can use a sprinkle of water for moisture.

Mix together base ingredients and spoon into a greased (use spray) cooking dish. Combine the topping mix and crumble over the base.

Bake at 350 degrees for 20 to 30 minutes or until golden brown. You can also cook this in the microwave—cooking times vary so keep an eye on it.

Serve with 1 scoop of vanilla nonfat sugar-free yogurt or Very Vanilla Sorbeto (page 259) for special occasions. Just as good with a cup of vanilla tea.

Cocoa Meringues

Minutes to Prepare: 10 ◆ Cooking Time: 2 hours ◆ Servings: 10 (4 per serving)

I'm obsessed with meringues and these little cookies fulfill the craving for something sweet without the guilt. They do have a little bit of sugar, but we all have those moments when we just need something yummy. I call these Heavenly Cookies because they are a lot lower in calories, free of fat, gluten, flours, and starch, and are made from minimal ingredients. The meringue options are limitless—so get creative and try topping them with crushed almonds that have been tossed in cinnamon and Stevia. For Christmas I like to top them with crushed candy canes.

3 egg white
1/3 cup sugar (superfine, if possible)
2 tablespoons unsweetened cocoa

1/8 teaspoon cream of tartar
1/4 teaspoon almond extract

Preheat oven to 200. Cover a baking sheet with parchment paper.

Place egg whites and cream of tartar in large bowl, beat with mixer at high speed until foamy. Add sugar, 1 tablespoon at a time, beating until stiff peaks form. Beat in extract.

Spoon mixture into pastry bag or zip lock plastic bag with 1 corner snipped to a ¼-inch-sized opening. Pipe 40 (1 inch round) mounds 1/4-inch apart onto prepared baking sheet. Bake at 200 for 2 hours.

Turn off oven, coo meringues in closed oven at least 1 hour.

Carefully remove meringues from paper and toss them with cocoa in zip-top plastic bag to coat.

Homemade Baked Cinnamon Apple Chips

Minutes to Prepare: 5 to 10 ◆ Cooking Time: 2 to 3 hours ◆ Servings: 4

Do you crave crunch? This one's for you. I can't help but devour these as soon as they are out of the oven. You can also make extra to take with you to work or when you travel. This is one of the most delicious ways get a serving of fruit in your day. As you know, apples are one of my top snack suggestions and make the Top Ten list of snacks on every diet on the planet from Atkins to Paleo. I cleaned up the usual version and made this one sugar-free, which not only makes this recipe better for your metabolism, but it also makes it a great snack for kids, too. It contains only two ingredients, so it's very simple. Make sure to use apples that have a great flavor to begin with, ones that you would enjoy eating raw. Otherwise the chips might turn out bitter and you'll be wondering why. I like to make the apple chips on a weekend morning so that they are ready for a late afternoon snack since it takes so long to dehydrate the apples in the oven. WARNING: These are addictive.

1 to 2 apples (I use Honey Crisp)   1 teaspoon cinnamon

Preheat oven to 200 degrees.

Using a sharp knife or mandolin, slice apples thinly. Discard seeds. Prepare a baking sheet with parchment paper and arrange apple slices on it without overlapping. Sprinkle cinnamon over apples.

Bake for approximately 1 hour, then flip. Continue baking for 1 to 2 hours, flipping occasionally, until the apple slices are no longer moist. Store in airtight container. The baking time varies, depending on your oven and how thick the apple slices were cut. You want to cut them as thinly as possible. Usually, mandolins work better for this sort of work, but I have found that the whole apple can be too wide for a mandolin. I use a sharp knife, which is why the thickness varies a teeny bit.

My Trick: I sprinkle a little metabolism-boosting vanilla Complete Protein powder to add sweetness instead of sugar.

HOMEMADE FROZEN STRAWBERRY POPS

Minutes to Prepare: 3 ◆ Freezing Time: 2 hours ◆ Servings: 4

Of course the best way to lose weight fast and enjoy a frozen treat is to freeze your Complete Protein Shake. But these more than do. Frozen pops are great to have around a house with kids (and all their friends). I love these in the summer when it's boiling outside; it's a delicious way to get more fluids in. I also love making these with Crystal Light Pink Lemonade or Peach Iced Tea, but this is the one that my kids love best and I like it because they are eating something that's good for them.

3 cups fat-free plain Greek yogurt   2 cups frozen unsweetened strawberries
2 teaspoons vanilla extract   2 tablespoons of honey or agave nectar, or Splenda

Combine yogurt, strawberries, vanilla extract, and sweetener of choice in blender. Process until smooth.

Pour the mixture into 4 ice-pop molds or paper cups. Place ice cream stick in the middle of each cup and freeze for 2 hours or until solid.

To serve, remove from molds or peel away paper cup.

Variation: For a truly decadent frozen pop, mix a frozen banana with a 1/2 scoop of chocolate Complete Protein powder. Unbelievably good.

ESPRESSO GRANITA

Minutes to Prepare: 10 ◆ Freezing Time: 2 hours or more ◆ Servings: 4

Forget driving the into town for a scoop of fattening ice cream that will set you back a half-day's worth of calories. Frozen granitas are just as satisfying as ice cream and very easy to make. Your metabolism and wallet will thank you as you'll save lots of calories and money. Unlike most versions of granitas this one is sugar-free and extremely low-calorie—it's practically free food.

2 cups espresso or very strong brewed coffee, warmed   1/2 cup of Splenda or Truvia
½ cup shaved dark chocolate   *light* whipped topping (optional)

Combine espresso or coffee with Splenda or Truvia and stir until dissolved. Pour mixture into shallow metal baking pan and place in freezer.

After 20 minutes, just as the mix begins to freeze, remove the pan from the freezer and use fork to scrape the ice crystals developing on the surface. Scraping will help you achieve a light, creamy granita rather than a chunky, icy one.

Return the pan to freezer and repeat this step every 30 minutes until granita is entirely frozen.

To serve, I scoop it into a chilled wine glass. For special occasions, I layer each serving alternating between granita and light whipped topping with chocolate shaving.

CPSIA information can be obtained at www.ICGtesting.com
Printed in the USA
BVOW10s0311170414

350859BV00001B/1/P